Medicinal Herb Handbook

An Herbal Application Guide
for Novice and Clinician
Through Simplified Herbal Remedy Descriptions

Feather Jones
Clinical Herbalist

LOTUS
PRESS

Published by:
Lotus Press
P.O. Box 325; Twin Lakes, WI 53181 USA

DISCLAIMER

This book is a reference work, not intended to diagnose, prescribe or treat. The information contained herein is in no way to be considered as a substitute for consultation with a licensed health-care professional. It is designed to provide information on traditional uses of herbs and historical folklore remedies.

For inquiries contact Lotus Press,
P.O. Box 325, Twin Lakes, WI 53181 U.S.A.
e-mail lotuspress@lotuspress.com
800-824-6396

Second Edition March 1999
Printed in the United States of America

ISBN 0-914955-87-x

Teach your children
what we have taught our children--
that the earth is our mother.
Whatever befalls the earth
befalls the sons and daughters of the earth.
If men spit upon the ground,
they spit upon themselves.

This we know.
The earth does not belong to us,
we belong to the earth.
This we know.
All things are connected
like the blood which unites one family.
All things are connected.

Whatever befalls the earth
befalls the sons and daughters of the earth.
We did not weave the web of life,
We are merely a strand in it.
Whatever we do to the web,
we do to ourselves. . .

Chief Seattle

TABLE OF CONTENTS

NP-*Not for use during pregnancy*

Medicinal Herb Handbook
Feather Jones, Clinical Herbalist

Introduction

Herbal medicine is finding a niche in the alternative health care field. Earth-centered values and global consciousness are taking the forefront in our resolve to heal the planet of its human-made diseases. A return to traditional plant therapy is becoming more mainstream as we recognize that pharmaceutical companies are disrupting third world cultures. Rainforest lands and what were once non-industrialized countries are being destroyed from the polluting wastes of this industry's manufacturing processes.

As herb buyers, we have an impact on global health and ecology. We can insist on buying only organically grown bulk herbs and herbal products and ask our health food stores to carry more of them. If you are buying wild harvested (wildcrafted) herbs and products, you may want to make sure they were ethically harvested. That means they were collected in the wild using conservative techniques that ensure maximum species preservation.* Many of our popular medicinals: Echinacea angustifolia, Lady's Slipper, Wild American Ginseng, and Golden Seal are inappropriately over harvested to the point of becoming threatened and endangered. Ask your retail stores and natural practitioners to provide you with enough information from the company selling wildcrafted herbs to get a feel for their ethical standards.

We can care for our health, support biological diversity and encourage corporate responsibility at the same time. Using herbal remedies manufactured by environmentally responsible companies is self-empowering, rewarding and helps to maintain a green planet. Our commitment to the earth is to maintain 'earth-centered' consciousness within our products and to honor native traditional values. This allows us to create an effortless flow in accordance with the laws of nature in our work place and our individual lives.

The information in this booklet is a collection of my clinical years of working with the plants, some of it is passed down generationally, some is from cultural uses world wide. Most is a harmonious mixture of experiences, research and ethnobotany, with no clear lines drawn as to ownership.

Some of the more technical information is based on human trials to the best of my knowledge, though animal models seem to find their way into herbal research as easily as pharmaceutical trials. I do not condone laboratory animal studies as it's barbaric, unethical and many times unreliable. A little known statistic: in 1989, there were 160,000 drug induced (iatrogenic) deaths reported in the US and approximately 20-40% of all drugs have proven side effects. All these pharmaceuticals went through rigorous animal studies before reaching the market. On the other hand, herbal medicine is self validated. Generations of usage have shown the safety and efficacy of knowledgeable and responsible administration.

This booklet is meant to guide you through simplified, to the point remedy descriptions of over 200 single and combination herbals. Each plant's descriptive value is based on the whole plant in it's entire natural state, (ie., root, flower, leaf, or seed) and not the isolated "active" constituent of a standardized product.

Standardization implies the measure of validity and quality is synonymous to chemical analysis. This is like saying only one part of the complex make up of a plant has any value. Somewhere along the way, we have lost sight of the concept of synergy. Herbal synergy means the whole plant is larger than the sum of it's parts. Whole plants are more than their specific constituents. They are multi-system wholistic medicines. As an herbalist, I've found it to be a great joy and honor over the years to connect with each plant, getting to know it's unique and subtle personality and characteristics. Just like people, they have myriad qualities and just like people, they are not single minded. You can't standardize people, nor should we desire to.

Many times a standardized product will be so strong, it more closely resembles a drug. As a drug, it may show side effects. Because Ginkgo is a vasodilator to the brain, some standardized Ginkgo products are causing occular hemorrhaging, bleeding from the eyes. That's too much blood to the head.

Healing the whole body vs. Disease

Herbs, like drugs, can be used to mask or chase symptoms around in the body. An herbalist though, sees the whole person from a constitutional perspective and treats the whole body. Herbal tonics are meant to strengthen and support a person's constitution, increasing their overall health and vitality, so disease, if it manifests at all, does not have to be so life threatening. An herbalist will also look to diet and nutrition, exercise, life style choices and a positive attitude having equally complimentary and essential therapeutic value. This is a wholistic and vitalistic approach not usually addressed in an allopathic treatment plan.

The human body is not single minded. One person who's over- stressed by an upcoming tax audit may have problems with gastric ulcers; another's nerves may become frayed and experience insomnia, laying awake at night trying to figure out how to balance the books. Another person's blood pressure may rise because they are in sympathetic mode, the old fight or flight mechanism we use when faced with constant challanges of crisis proportions. The sympathetic nervous system vasoconstricts the peripheral arterioles and capillary beds shunting a higher volume of blood to the heart, elevating blood pressure.

If you mask a symptom, you halt the body's ability to manifest it's imbalance and recreate equilibrium on it's own. By repeatedly doing this, you may drive the disorder deeper into the body. It will eventually surface with a more serious pathology with probable immune compromise. Herbal therapies can be used to help aid the body by supporting the vital force which strengthens whole body function, smoothly adapting the individual to daily stresses without over-responding with an ulcer, or other symptomatic result. Herbs can even help restore a person's sense of well being through feeling nourished and balanced.

As popular magazine ads and television commercials will tell you, when your child has a cough, you should give a cough suppressant. With this accomplished, you no longer have to listen to the cough. This may be seen as an analogy to a building fire when the smoke alarm goes off. Should we only then cut off the alarm? We would no longer have to hear it.

Coughing is a natural reflex of the body to eliminate excess mucus, infections, allergens and bacteria from the respiratory tract. The more vitalistic approach would be to give expectorant herbs that help facilitate the upward movement of mucus out of the bronchioles. Expectorants support and stimulate mucous membranes to create a more productive cough and strengthen the system while doing it.

Another example is a fever that accompanies the flu. The first impulse when a person has a fever is to bring the temperature down. A fever is the body's way of burning out the toxins making you sick. By suppressing this, the body must again find another avenue of elimination. The herbal strategy here would be to help support the fever by allowing the blood to stay hot, yet cool the body down. Herbal diaphoretics can accomplish this by opening the pores of the skin, allowing the individual to sweat, releasing excess heat and toxins.

Herbal Combinations

The middle section of this book contains some of my favorite and most effective formulas. Some are herbal hand me downs, some are from the old National Formulary and most are ones I created myself for lack of something better out there.

When herbs are compounded into formulas, they may achieve a more focused action. There is always a main herb or herbs of similar intent guiding the directive of the formula. Other herbs are added to support their goal. Some formulas have gentle, buffering herbs added to them to soften harsh herbal actions not desired in the outcome. Others may have warming, stimulating sattelite herbs to increase the intensity of the main herb to help drive it deeper into congested areas of the body that the main herb alone would not be able to accomplish.

Cautions and Considerations

1. Herbs that are considered safe by many may not be appropriate during pregnancy. Deep liver cleansing herbs and laxatives are ones to be especially mindful of. I have used the symbol *N/P (not for pregnancy)* after each herb described.

2. Be mindful, herbs may present overt drug reactions if mixed with pharmaceuticals or any medical treatments. Always check with a physican and clinical herbalist first.

3. If you are buying bulk herbs, you can many times check the strength of the herb by it's taste, smell and color, meaning there should be some. For example, Alfalfa leaf should smell slightly like new mowed hay and with Echinacea root you should taste the familiar tingle on the tongue.

4. When buying wildcrafted herbs, find out if the company complies with ethical harvesting practices. Black Cohosh, a popular herb used in menopause all over Europe, only grows in the eastern forest of the US. To date, according to industry sources, no one is commercially growing this plant. It's overharvested and will end up like Golden Seal on the CITES endangered plant list if we don't create accountability with our manufacturers now. Retailers should have a company's specs on file.

5. For herbs to act quickly, they need to be taken on an empty stomach.

6. The concept "if a little is good, more is better"; usually doesn't translate to herbal remedies, particularly extracts and tinctures that are already concentrated.

7. If the remedy makes you sick, take less or throw it away.

Hopefully this booklet will whet your appetite and encourage you to continue your search for more knowledge about medicinal plants and their benefits. When the opportunity arises, take an herb walk and get a first handed acquaintance with the plants.

To your health

> Feather Jones
> Lyons, Colorado

* You can obtain a list of ethical harvesters of medicinal plants from the Rocky Mountain Herbalist Coalition, P.O. Box 165, Lyons, CO 80540

If you are interested in studying herbs and the practice of herbalism you can contact the Rocky Mountain Center for Botanical Studies. They will provide you with information about their certification program or workshops. You may contact them at:

> RMCBS
> P.O. Box 19254,
> Boulder, CO 80308-2254
> rmcbs@indra.com
> www.herbschool.com
> or call (303) 442-6861.

SINGLE PLANTS

Agrimony *(Agrimonia striata/eupatoria)* This plant is useful in urinary tract infections and over-active or hypermetabolic liver as in chemotherapy or drug excess.

Aletris *(Aletris farinosa)* As a gynecological tonic, it aids digestion and low back pain associated with pelvic prolapse or congestion.

Alfalfa *(Medicago sativa)* This nutritive herb has a high mineral content that is easily digestible, particularly calcium, vitamin K, and folic acid; stimulates lactation while increasing the quality of breast milk.

Angelica *(Angelica spp.)* Used in weak digestion; as an anti-spasmodic, it prevents uterine and intestinal cramping and regulates menses due to hormonal balancing properties. (NP)

Arnica *(Arnica cordifolia/latifolia)* For external use only; it works as a liniment for joint inflam-mation, sprains and sore muscles to decrease swelling and bruising; and helps with neuromuscular tone as in arthritis.

Aspen *(Populus tremuloides)* As an anti-inflammatory and fever reducer, it has aspirin-like effects without the usual stomach irritation.

Astragalus *(Astragalus membranicus)* As an immune system builder and strengthener, this herb is a deep tonic that replenishes bone marrow.

Baptisia *(Baptisia tinctoria)* Having blood cleansing properties for septic conditions and degenera-tive diseases, it will stimulate metabolism of waste products and cellular repair. USE WITH CARE. (NP)

Barberry *(Berberis fendleri)* Good for sluggish liver, gallstones, herpes, ulcers and jaundice; it will lower fevers, inflammations and blood pressure; acts as intestinal strengthener and laxative. (NP)

Bayberry *(Myrica cerifera)* Topically and as a gargle or douche, it shrinks swollen tissues in gin-givitis and tonsillitis, vaginitis and discharges. Internally it increases systolic and diastolic pressure.

Benzoin *(Styrax benzoin)* This herb softens up bronchiole mucus, giving it expectorating quali-ties; makes a nice steam in the vaporizer.

Betony *(Pedicularis spp.)* As an effective sedative for hyper-active children and adults, it relaxes the skeletal muscles; decreases muscular pain and relaxes muscle spasm.

Black Cohosh *(Cimicifuga racemosa)* As an anti-spasmodic, it works on ovarian neuralgia with shooting pain or sharp menstrual cramps; a specific for boggy feeling in the pelvis during menses; aids menopause process by stimulating circulation while sedating central nervous system. (NP)

Black Haw *(Viburnum prunifolium)* For painful periods, clotting and low back pain in menses; it will increase scanty flow and allay a threatened miscarriage.

Black Walnut *(Juglans nigra)* This herb helps with oil-soluble vitamins and B12 absorption asso-ciated with illeo-cecal inflammations; for intestinal flora imbalances, it tones the GI tract. Works well for diarrhea, constipation, giardia and dysentery. As an anti-fungal, it may help in yeast infec-tions.

Blessed Thistle *(Cnicus benedictus)* Having bitter properties, it stimulates digestive activity and is used to treat gastritis and peptic ulcers; this herb also helps supply estrogen aid to a deficient sys-tem and stimulates milk let down. (NP)

Bloodroot *(Sanguinaria canadensis)* In small doses, it is a stimulant and expectorant for a dry irritating non-productive cough, helping clear the bronchials of mucus. In large doses, it is a depressant, causing headache and nausea. In poisonous doses, it can cause respiratory failure. USE CAUTIOUSLY. Contains anti-fungal properties with external use. (NP)

Blueberry *(Bilberry) (Vaccinium myrtillus)* Good for tired eyes from computer stress as it regenerates rhodopsin (retinal purple); also stimulates urine output and strengthens the heartbeat.

Blue Cohosh *(Caulophyllum thalictroides)* Helpful in uterine infections as it increases excess fluid drainage; it will initiate a late period and decrease cramping and spotting at the end of a period. (NP)

Blue Flag *(Iris missouriensis)* Called a liver lymphatic, it gets natural oils to the skin and is good mixed with other herbs for blood toxicity; a strong diaphoretic (increases perspiration) and powerful liver stimulant; it will increase the metabolism and assimilation of complex foods for deficient body types. (NP)

Blue Vervain *(Verbena hastata)* This mellowing herb cools out acid indigestion where heartburn is present and slows down hyperfunctions; good for kids sick with the flu and agitated. (NP)

Boneset *(Eupatorium perfoliatum)* As a fever reducer and pain modifier, it can be of service in flu symptoms where there's deep seated achy muscular and joint pain; as an expectorant, it will help facilitate the movement of mucus out of the lungs where there is a weakened cough with lots of secretions but a lack of power to cough it out.

Brickellia *(Prodigiosa) (Brickellia grandiflora)* A specific for adult onset insulin-resistant diabetes by decreasing the liver's overproduction of glucose (decreasing gluconeogenesis).

Buchu *(Barosma serratifolia)* As a urinary disinfectant, it is helpful in chronic cystitis or urethritis in an acid environment, due to colon bacteria invasion.

Bugleweed *(Lycopus americanus)* As a constitutional strengthener, this herb is for hyperthyroid states and over-rapid GI transit time; irregular heartbeat and insomnia.

Burdock *(Arctium minus)* Alkalinizes and eliminates toxins in the bloodstream; best for chronic acne and psoriasis; used in prolapsed uterus and gout with excess uric acid production. Will cool yet strengthen a hot liver with excess anabolic stress.

Calendula *(Calendula officinalis)* Used for pus filled infections and ulcerations as a topical application; with glycerine as a douche, it may be used for vaginitis, cervitis, and non-specific discharges; it decreases the scarring process and promotes healing.

Cascara Sagrada *(Rhamnus purshiana)* Used in chronic constipation, indigestion and hemorrhoids; it is helpful in gallstones and liver ailments. (NP)

Catnip *(Nepeta cataria)* This gentle herb is excellent for children and infants with colic and teething pain; digestive pains, feverish colds and nervous headaches.

Cat's Claw *(Uncaria tomentosa)* An immune system enhancer, it has found use in arthritis, cancer, allergies and systemic candida; also reported to synergistically work with AZT for HIV and AIDS, while reducing side effects of chemotherapy; also increases circulation and inhibits formation of plaque and blood clots in the brain, heart and arteries, lowering blood pressure and helping with thrombosis; as an anti-oxidant, anti-viral and anti-tumor, it helps the body fight infections better. (NP)

Cayenne *(Capsicum spp.)* It builds up resistance at the beginning of a cold; helpful in stomach and lower bowel pains; improves circulation to extremities; good liniment for rheumatism and arthritis. Use sparingly.

Celandine, Greater *(Chelidonium majus)* Finds usefulness in asthmatic symptoms and digestive problems including colitis; liver congestion. (NP)

Chamomile *(Matricaria spp.)* Helps with acid indigestion and gas from food fermentation, decreasing the ability of the nerves to repolarize; may also help in morning sickness and general nausea.

Chaparral *(Larrea spp.)* Tones the liver and increases dietary fat metabolism; treats rheumatism, malignant growths, and radiation poisoning; pulls heavy metals out of the body.

Chaparro Amargosa *(Castela emoryi)* Especially useful in amoebic dysentery and giardiasis, it acts as an active inhibitor of all intestinal protozoa. Used as a preventative when traveling, it will limit infections before they occur as well as after the fact. A secondary treatment for candida and bacterial enteritis.

ChasteTree *(Vitex agnus-castus)* As a tonic and normalizer to the reproductive organs, it stimulates progesterone where there is deficiency or will act to normalize hormone production in dysmenorrhea, PMS symptoms and menopausal changes. (NP)

Chickweed *(Stellaria media)* Used in rheumatism where the pains shift alot; also it helps control dietary fat metabolism.

Cinnamon *(Cinnamomum cassia)* Used as a hemostat, it is serviceable in hemorrhaging and excess menses bleeding; being astringent, it is also useful for diarrhea and excess gas.

Cleavers *(Galium aparine)* A simple diuretic, it is used for lower urinary tract inflammations with fluid accumulation; as a gentle blood purifier, it corrects lymphatic swellings.

Clematis *(Clematis spp.)* Used in classic migraines and cluster headaches; nervous tics from stress associated with too low blood pressure and food allergen headaches. (NP)

Comfrey *(Symphytum officinale)* Useful in broken bones, sprains and damaged tendons; it will stimulate respiratory organs and eliminates expectoration; helpful in arthritis, stomach problems, ulcerated tonsils, abscesses, and wounds; makes an excellent mouthwash for bleeding gums; good for anemia and diarrhea. With extended use, it may irritate the liver. (NP)

Corn Silk *(Zea mays)* Used for painful urination to soothe the membranes, increase urinary output and dilute solid waste.

Cotton Root *(Gossypium thurberi)* For scanty crampy menstruation associated with dragging pelvic pains and backache; traditionally used as an abortifacient, it seems to increase receptor sites on oxytocin sensitive cells, thereby causing uterine contractions. (NP)

Cow Parsnip *(Heracleum sphondylium)* *Dry* — for gas, acid indigestion and persistent nausea; as an anti-spasmodic for the GI tract, it may help with spastic colitis and cramping.

   Fresh — topically used as a nerve irritant/stimulant in recent paralysis; added to bath water, it exaggerates and excites the nerves.

Cramp Bark *(Viburnum opulus)* As a uterine sedative and tonic, it is good for menses cramps, leg cramps and mild convulsions; will help with over-irritability of the uterus preventing miscarriages as it quiets down contractions.

Damiana *(Turnera diffusa)* Used as a natural upper for nervous and sexual debility, it will revitalize the reproductive system in both sexes. As a hormone balancer, it strengthens the ovum in women and increases sperm count in men. (NP)

Dandelion *(Taraxacum officinale)* *Fresh whole plant* (spring harvest) — As an electrolyte balancer, this is our best diuretic because it doesn't deplete potassium, it is good for kidney inflammations. This "spring tonic" has blood cleansing effects.

   Dry or fresh root (autumn harvest) — It is a mild laxative for habitual constipation; good to cool out excess liver functions.

Desert Willow *(Chilopsis linearis)* Acting similarly to Pau D'Arco, it inhibits some fungal infections and has been used for many immune system-related problems. It seems to control candida infections at the upper and lower ends of the intestinal tract and is especially significant for after antibiotic therapy or anti-inflammatory drugs that alter the gut bacteria.

Devil's Claw *(Harpagophytum procumbens)* A good first approach for rheumatoid and osteo-arthritis as an anti-inflammatory and acts to decrease blood fats, cholesterol and uric acid levels; also good for gout and adrenal cortical problems.

Devil's Club *(Oplopanax horridum)* Used to help control blood sugar levels in adult onset, insulin-resistant diabetes; a Ginseng-like adaptogen that can be especially useful for stressed individuals with dry skin; a reliable expectorant to create a productive cough. (NP)

Dogbane *(Apocynum cannabinum)* Internally, this cardiac stimulant should be used with caution; in small doses it acts as a vasoconstrictor, slowing and strengthening the heartbeat and increasing blood pressure. Externally, it stimulates circulation and nerve repair applied to referred pain areas, such as sciatica, uterine pain and spinal cord injuries. As a hair rinse, it stimulates hair follicle growth. SHOULD BE PHYSICIAN ADMINISTERED ONLY. (NP)

Dong Quai *(Angelica sinensis cured)* As a reproductive hormone balancer, it can correct urethritis, prostatitis and cervicitis associated with constipation and poor estrogen production; helpful in PMS symptoms by increasing receptor sites on hormone-sensitive cells to steroid hormones; anti-spasmodic. (NP)

Echinacea *(Echinacea angustifolia)* This blood purifier stimulates white blood cell count at an area of infection; its anti-viral, antibacterial, and anti-biotic properties stimulate quick tissue repair. Good for colds, flus, infections and fevers.

Elder flower *(Sambucus spp.)* This plant acts as a fever reducer by both resetting the fever control mechanism within the brain and stimulates sweating. With equal parts of Peppermint and Yarrow, this remedy has been used since olden times.

Elecampane *(Inula helenium)* A remedy for chronic and persistent coughs where appetite is reduced, as an expectorant it stimulates the expulsion of mucus. It improves mucus membrane tone throughout the whole body and stimulates appetite and general well-being.

Eucalyptus *(Eucalyptus globulus)* This herb may be used as a steam inhalation for its antiseptic and expectorating effects in bronchitis and influenza to relieve congestion. It is also serviceable in sluggish urinary tract infections of a chronic nature.

Eyebright *(Euphrasia officinalis)* Internally, it shrinks swollen sinuses in hay fever. As a rinse, it strengthens the tensile structure of the eyes making it good for eye inflammations and eye strain.

False Unicorn *(Chamaelirium luteum)* As a uterine tonic, this herb provides building material to form estrogen, also a specific for delayed and absent menstruation; it is useful in some threatened miscarriages associated with nervous irritability and periodic contractions. For menopausal symptoms associated with pelvic sluggishness and a sense of pressure with bladder irritability, value can be found. (NP)

Fennel *(Foeniculum spp.)* The aromatic oils act as a carminative to expel gas, stomach cramping and intestinal colic. It is also mildly calming to coughs and colds causing amenorrhea. It will increase lactation in nursing mothers.

Feverfew *(Chrysanthemum parthenium)* A reputation in the treatment of migraines, it acts as an anti-inflammatory and anti-spasmodic by opposing prostaglandin action. It may also help arthritis in acute inflammatory stages as well as painful periods with sluggish menses flow. (NP)

Fireweed *(Epilobium augustifolia)* As an astringent to stomach and intestinal tract, it is serviceable for diarrhea and the cramping associated with it; it is anti-spasmodic to colic, hiccoughs and spasms. A specific with Peppermint for summer diarrhea in kids.

Fringetree *(Chionanthus virginicus)* A remedy to aid liver congestion with gall bladder inflammation and gall stones excretion by a dilation of the hepatic duct, it will increase the flow of bile; used in hepatitis associated with liver enlargement and useful in poor fat metabolism due to faulty digestion.

Garlic *(Allium sativa)* When used in hypertension, it lowers cholesterol and triglyceride levels and inhibits platelet aggregation; as an anti-microbial it acts on bacteria, viruses and intestinal parasites.

Gentian *(Swertia radiata)* Taken as a bitter tonic, it will increase digestive enzymes and stimulate bile excretion to increase assimilation of dietary proteins and fats. It also stimulates appetite and may help with chronic flatulence.

Ginger *(Zingiber officinale)* For intestinal cramping and gas, indigestion; useful in cold fingers and toes in a cold climate; will cause sweating in a dry fever with chills, this herb has a pleasant spicy warming taste that dispels nausea in morning and motion sickness.

Ginkgo *(Ginkgo biloba)* This plant enhances mental abilities and increases concentration, aptitude, memory and alertness. It may be helpful in Alzheimer's disease by alleviating depression. It increases oxygen to the brain and regulates neurotransmitters and helps to make brain metabolism more efficient. Possible immune cell suppressant to benefit allergies and asthma. (NP)

Ginseng, American *(Panax quinquefolium)* Traditionally recommended for use in nervous exhaustion, it will nourish and tonify the adrenals, normalize blood pressure and decrease blood cholesterol. Labeled as an adaptogen, it will help the body to modify stress levels and strengthen the constitution. (NP)

Golden Rod *(Solidago spathulata)* This gentle and safe remedy relieves cramping with gas, a specific for kidney stones and obstructions or inflammation/ulceration in the bladder; tonic, soothing and healing to urinary tract disorders, helps to regenerate and rebuild kidneys.

Golden Seal *(Hydrastis canadensis)* With some of the main properties being only alcohol soluble, this root will stimulate mucus membrane secretion. As a powerful tonic to these tissues, it may alleviate gastritis, ulceration, colitis and some hay fever symptoms. Its antibiotic properties make it useful in cold symptoms. (NP)

Gotu Kola *(Centella asiatica)* As a cerebral stimulant, it carries nutrients for transport to the brain and rejuvenates neural synapses to help with poor memory and sluggish brain activity; for pruritis, combine with Skullcap and Oregon Grape as it will improve skin quality and calm the central nervous system.

Gravel Root *(Eupatorium purpureum)* As a diuretic, this plant will help prevent the precipitation of kidney stones and allows a free elimination of urates and uric acid crystals. A specific to sluggish prostate and cystitis with mucus discharge.

Grindelia *(Grindelia squarrosa)* With tonic effects on the lungs and kidneys, its stimulating action makes it useful as an expectorant to cough up obstinate catarrh; used in certain asthmas to dilate bronchioles and decrease chest constriction. For the urinary tract, it is mildly diuretic. Externally (fresh only) it can be applied to poison ivy and skin rashes to cool, soothe and prevent itching.

Green Tea *(camellia sinensia)* Strong flavonoid content gives this plant antioxidant proerties defending the body against free radicals and supporting the immune system. Reduces LDL serium levels and can keep blood sugar levels from rising, even though it's a nervous system stimulant similar to caffeine.

Guarana *(Paullinia cupana)* As a caffeine plant and central nervous system stimulant, it will increase neural and circulatory tone which may be needed in chronic diseases and convalescence; as a mood elevator, it produces a gaiety and is aphrodisiac. Least likely of all caffeine plants to cause anxiety.

Hawthorne *(Crataegus succulenta)* This plant has the ability of imparting muscular tone to cardiac action, making each beat count; as a heart tonic it is good for myocarditis and nervous heart problems including palpitations.

Hops *(Humulus lupulus)* A safe sedative for children and adults to promote sleep and control nervousness and nervous stomach problems related to faulty starch digestion. As a mild pain killer, it finds success in dysmenorrhea.

Horehound (*Marrubium vulgare*) An effective expectorant for dry hacking and unproductive cough; a respiratory sedative by relaxing and dilating bronchioles, it may be useful in certain asthmas; a syrup remedy for children.

Horse Chestnut (*Aesculus hippocastanum*) An astringent and tonic to the circulatory system, it strengthens and tones the veins and may be used in varicosities, hemorrhoids and phlebitis. (NP)

Horseradish (*Armoracia rusticana*) A stimulant to the digestive process to expel gas and cramping; it can be used in early stages of a cold as a circulatory mover; as a steam inhalant, it will loosen up tight mucus in the lungs.

Horsetail (*Equisetum arvense*) Due to its high silica content, it finds usefulness in emphysema, asthma and kidney disorders as it stabilizes scar tissue; strengthens tissues high in elastin properties like alveolar sacs within the lungs and nephron tubules within the kidneys.

Hyssop (*Hyssopus officinalis*) As a respiratory anti-viral and anti-spasmodic for croupy coughs, bronchitis and asthma; will bring on sweating with dry skin and a fever; a relaxing nervine for petit mal and anxiety states.

Inmortal (*Asclepias asperula*) As a bronchial dilator and stimulant to lymph drainage in the lungs, it's a good medicine for asthma, pleurisy and bronchitis. As a mild, reliable cardiac tonic to congestive heart disorders, it relieves pressure on the heart valve. A strong diaphoretic and menses stimulant. (NP)

Juniper (*Juniperus communis*) Useful in sluggish urinary tract disorders of a chronic nature and not for hot acute inflammation; a diuretic and stimulant to the stomach for stressed out digestive functions, it will increase HCL secretion. (NP)

Kava Kava (*Piper methysticum*) It has a stimulating effect on the urinary tract, the GI tract and the central nervous system, it is used as a diuretic, and appetizer and tonic to the GI tract promoting better dietary assimilation and produces a feeling of well-being.

Kelp (*Nereocystis luetkeana*) Because of its iodine binding ability in the thyroid, it acts as a radiation antagonist; an excellent mineral replacer for calcium and other important nutrients.

Kola Nut (*Cola nitida*) A caffeine plant that stimulates the entire cerebrum minimizing fatigue and promoting alertness; like coffee, not to be used extensively due to adrenal stress and exhaustion but periodically it will find value in neuromuscular hypofunction from long illnesses and depression.

Kudzu (*Pueraria lobata*) Used for alcohol addiction, it acts as a long term tonic, reducing blood pressure, elevated blood sugar, migraine headaches and stomach acidity.

Lavender (*Lavendula officinalis*) A great carminative in cases of nervous indigestion, gas, nausea and cramping; used as an inhalant to relieve some headaches; in the old days, it was part of a compound "smelling salts" and makes a good adjunct herb in a soothing syrup for children.

Lemon Balm (*Melissa officinalis*) A neural relaxant, it lowers the stress response and acts as a mood elevator in depressive states; an anti-spasmodic, it blocks nerve impulses and acts as a general mild sedative; also shown to have anti-viral effects in herpes, reducing the pain and shortening the outbreak. (NP)

Licorice (*Glycyrrhiza glabra*) With a soothing influence upon gastric mucosa, it's an excellent remedy for peptic and duodenal ulcerations, chronic bronchitis, arthritic symptoms and chronic constipation. Used for adrenal exhaustion as a strengthener to that organ's system. (NP)

Lily of the Valley (*Convallaria majalis*) Like digitalis as a cardiac tonic but less toxic, it will promote regular heart action and increase blood pressure in hypotensive cases; with Echinacea, it is reportedly useful in endocarditis — SHOULD BE PHYSICIAN ADMINISTERED ONLY. (NP)

Lobelia (*Lobelia inflata*) In moderate doses it will relax the lungs and dilate bronchioles; in overdoses it paralyzes the cerebrospinal centers and will cause nausea and a drop in blood pressure; in reasonable doses it is an anti-spasmodic and finds service in bronchial asthma.

Lomatium *(Lomatium dissectum)* Antiviral to respiratory infections being of service in sore throats and congestion; too much may cause a rash that is self limiting and part of the body's cleansing response as it opens the pores of the skin. (NP)

Ma Huang *(Ephedra vulgaris)* Because of its stimulating action with extended use, it will deplete the adrenal reserves, but for temporary relief it is beneficial in hay fever, sinus congestion and allergy induced asthma.

Maravilla *(Mirabilis multiflorum)* As an appetite suppressant, it relieves hunger pangs by anesthetizing the stomach lining and allows one to go longer between meals.

Marshmallow *(Althea officinalis)* A soothing agent to inflammations of the mouth, stomach, intestines, kidneys and bladder; also an astringent to these tissues and vaginal mucosa; an excellent respiratory syrup for sore throats. The polysaccharides found in this plant may be similar to the immune-stimulating properties found in Echinacea.

Matarique *(Cacalia decomposita)* It decreases the amount of insulin necessary in diabetes; a specific for non-compliance adult onset diabetes, it works on cell membrane permeability to blood sugar. (NP)

Milk Thistle *(Silybum marianum)* It is a liver protectant from chemical damage and improves liver function as a cell regenerator; an antidote to Amonita mushroom poisoning; prevents free radical damage as in cirrhosis and chronic hepatitis.

Mormon Tea *(Ephedra torreyana)* Serves a similar function to Ma Huang but less of a stimulant to the heart, blood pressure and pulse rate; a source of silica makes it good for mild kidney infections and osteoporosis. It's a bronchial dilator increasing breathing capacity in asthmatic conditions and hay fever by shrinking swollen membranes.

Motherwort *(Leonurus cardiaca)* Its mild vaso-dilating effects are employed in menses cramps associated with a delayed flow or scanty menstruation; its nervine properties find benefit in PMS and some menopausal symptoms; used post-partum, it helps to drain the uterus and prevent infections. (NP)

Mullein *(Verbascum thapsus)* A respiratory relaxant and bronchial dilator, it expands the airways allowing freer breathing; it will arrest paroxysmal uncontrollable coughs finding relief in whooping cough, bronchitis and asthma. The oil may be used in earaches as an anti-bacterial and pain killer.

Myrrh Gum *(Commiphora molmol)* Makes a good anti-bacterial gargle for sores in mouth, gums and throat; increases white blood cell count. Externally, it binds with squamous cells to form a tanning film for tightening boggy tissues; prevents hyaluronidase and keeps tissues from breaking down and may find use in some auto-immune disorders.

Nettles *(Urtica gracilis)* Its diuretic action flushes the urinary tract of accumulated waste and helps to replace lost electrolytes; being high in assimilable iron, calcium and chlorophyll makes it an excellent nutritional supplement; good adjunct in menopause due to high calcium assimilation.

Oat Seed *(Avena sativa/fatua)* The milky unripe seeds contain anti-inflammatory and tonic properties that are nourishing to the nervous system; good for coming off drugs and addictions, it will strengthen and ground the individual; great for children.

Ocotillo *(Fouqueria splendens)* It is good for glandular and lymphatic swellings and intestinal blockages or adhesions from surgery; chronic pleurisy and water on the lungs, should be used with facilitator herbs. (NP)

Oregon Grape Root *(Mahonia repens)* This blood purifier is beneficial in skin conditions such as acne, eczema, herpes and psoriasis; useful in constipation, rheumatism and chronic liver malfunctions of a deficient nature. (NP)

Oshá *(Ligusticum porteri)* As a bronchial dilator and expectorant and anti-viral agent, it is useful in respiratory infections, colds, flus, sore throats, smoking and dry membranes, it stimulates resoftening and protects alveolar sac integrity; a strong diaphoretic. (NP)

Pansy *(Viola tricolor)* As a child's remedy, it contains methylsalicylates that decrease inflammation, reduce a fever and have a positive effect on jaundice; called an herbal aspirin and gentle sedative.

Partridge Berry *(Squaw Vine) (Mitchella repens)* As a tonic, it is recommended for the last few weeks of pregnancy for an easier childbirth; with Cramp Bark, it is useful in difficult periods.

Passion Flower *(Passiflora incarnata)* The anti-spasmodic, sedative and mood elevating qualities have value in nervous insomnia without giving a narcotic hangover, as well as neuralgia; used in asthma combinations and seizures.

Pau D'Arco *(Tabebuia impeteginosa)* Used in treating systemic and yeast infections, as it inhibits candida enzymes from reproducing; also has an anti-oxidant effect and will increase red blood cell count.

Pennyroyal *(Hedeoma pulegioides)* As an anti-spasmodic, it is useful in flatulent colic, painful menses, and abdominal cramps, and to help break up colds. Taken hot it will increase sweating and may be useful in high fevers. (NP)

Pipsissewa *(Chimaphila umbellata)* This plant stimulates removal of wastes in the kidneys and flushes the urinary tract, it also is a tonic and anti-bacterial to the system.

Plantain *(Plantago major)* Being high in chlorophyll, this plant is an excellent wound healer, for abrasions, rashes and insect bites; internally, it is healing to GI tract inflammations from stomach ulcers to dysentery and septicemic conditions of the blood.

Pleurisy *(Asclepias tuberosa)* It is good for dry coughs and congestion as it will remoisten the lungs making expectoration easier, will also increase sweating and can be used for colds with fevers and flu symptoms. Will relieve difficulty in breathing, bronchitis and pleurisy. (NP)

Poke *(Phytolacca americana)* In conservative doses, it is an excellent alterative and lymphatic stimulant to clear up over acid bloodstream; will detoxify the body after a protracted illness; a specific for lymphatic swellings, it works synergistically in combinations. (NP)

Poleo Mint *(Mentha arvensis)* Being stronger than peppermint as a diaphoretic to stimulate sweating, this plant works well with Elder to break a fever; and as a stomatic, it is useful in colic and stomachache to relax the muscle coats. (NP)

Prickly Ash *(Xanthoxylum americanum)* For signs of poor circulation such as cold extremities, varicose veins and chilblains, it is a stimulating tonic, used as a carminative, it will increase digestive juices and warm the stomach and will promote the appetite.

Prickly Poppy *(Argemone hispida)* Externally used for heat rash, hives and other eruptions; also for sunburn to relieve pain; internally, as a sedative to bring on sleep and reduce pain.

Propolis *(Propolis — Aspen gathered)* This resin contains astringent properties making it useful in dysentery, sore throats, tonsillitis, diarrhea, edema, blistering; for food allergies by blocking protein enzyme production (by blocking the breakdown of gels to mush) and damaged tissues; helpful in auto-immune diseases. Topically, sterilizes skin disorders and speeds healing time of herpes blisters. Should be lead free. Not for those with bee allergies.

Pulsatilla *(Pulsatilla patens)* As a sedative to produce a restful sleep, it may be employed for drug abuse and feelings of overwrought; for knowing you are going to over react to a situation, but can't help yourself; emotional fragility and exaggeration. (NP)

Quassia *(Picranea excelsa)* As an amoebocide, it can be used to treat giardia, dysentery, pinworms, and poor gastrointestinal function in general. (NP)

Raspberry *(Rubus idaeus)* This uterine tonic is used for excess menses bleeding and during pregnancy to prevent spotting; will cut down on postpartum bleeding and is mildly laxative.

Red Clover *(Trifolium pratense)* Contains a high mineral content and has mild sedative effects on children; a good maintenance and nutritive herb in hepatitis and mononucleosis or any chronic disease state.

Red Root *(Ceanothus fendleri)* As a lymphatic strengthener and supporter to the immune system, it can be used for tonsillitis, sore throat, enlarged lymph nodes, non-fibrous cysts, enlarged spleen, menstrual hemorrhage, nosebleed and sinus inflammations; also used as a gargle due to its astringent qualities.

Reishi Mushroom *(Ganoderma lucidum)* Normalizes high blood pressure and decreases effects of stress on the cardiovascular system; improves the flow of blood to the head, it enhances memory and promotes overall vitality and longevity.

Rosemary *(Rosmarinus officinalis)* Called the "herb of remembrance," it acts to improve circulation to the head; contains anti-oxidant and preserving properties; internally may be used to normalize blood pressure and strengthen capillaries in the brain; relieves debility and depression associated with nervous disorders.

Sage *(Salvia leucophylla)* Can be used in ulcer formulas to decrease hypersecretions in stomach; it is antiseptic and diaphoretic to increase sweating in fevers and flus; will decrease lactation, not recommended for nursing mothers.

Saw Palmetto *(Serenoa serrulata)* To reduce inflammation, it is serviceable in chronic prostatitis from constant irritation; it corrects pelvic sluggishness and will control mucus discharges; may be used to control incontinence in children and adults.

Schisandra *(Schisandra chinensis)* With a protective effect on liver cells and a non-specific balancing effect on metabolism, it decreases fatigue and increases natural resistance for the immune system; intensifies mental activity and alertness; stabilizes blood pressure and tones the cardiovascular system; adjusts stomach acid and lowers blood sugar levels.

Shepherd's Purse *(Capsella bursa-pastoris)* The fresh extract is valuable in bladder irritations associated with bleeding and phosphate deposits; also used for menstrual hemorrhaging and placental delivery in childbirth. (NP)

Siberian Ginseng *(Eleutherococcus senticosis)* An adaptogen, meaning it increases performance, stamina and endurance levels, increases the body's resistance to stress, increases mental alertness and provides a normalizing action on metabolism; shows some protective ability to radiation toxicity. (NP)

Skullcap *(Scutellaria lateriflora)* Useful in insomnia, fear, nervous and migraine headaches to slow down nerve synapsual speed and decrease end organ irritability from hypersensitivity; may be helpful in sciatica, transitory pain in MS and neuralgia.

Spikenard *(Aralia racemosa)* The roots of this plant contain phytosterols that resemble Ginseng in neural-hormonal effect; will buffer stress references in the brain; makes a strong reliable expectorant in acute bronchitis and elderly smokers.

St. John's Wort *(Hypericum perforatum)* Being high in bioflavinoids, it can be used externally and internally to increase capillary integrity in problems with varicosities such as hemorrhoids, varicose veins and easy bleeders; internally acts as an anti-depressant (mao inhibitor) and a remedy for the blues; contains anti-viral and anti-bacterial properties good in ear infections, externally helps in nerve damage and inflammations along the spinal cord.

Stillingia *(Stillingia sylvatica)* Makes an excellent respiratory syrup for dry hacking coughs; as a lymph drainer it works well on skin and fungal infections, dermatitis and eczema to clarify swollen toxic tissues. USE CONSERVATIVELY INTERNALLY. (NP)

Storksbill *(Erodium cicutarium)* As a mild uterine hemostat, it can be used after childbirthing to cut down on postpartum bleeding to prevent secondary infections; it is mildly astringent to urinary tract infections and will acidify the urine to normal.

Thuja *(Thuja occidentalis)* Highly anti-fungal, it is effective in skin problems with ringworm, jock itch, athlete's foot and candidas; works in urinary tract infections as it retards bacterial growth, use only short term as it may irritate kidneys; good in amoebic dysentery and giardia. (NP)

Toadflax *(Linaria vulgaris)* Best for chronic liver irritations and hepatitis flareups; useful for workers around industrial solvents, painters and mechanics. (NP)

Usnea *(Usnea spp.)* Being similar to penicillin, it can be used for gram positive bacterial infections such as strep, staph, impetigo, tuberculosis or yeast but does not effect intestinal flora.

Uva Ursi *(Arctostaphylos uva ursi)* A specific for nephritis, cystitis and urethritis and all urinary tract bacterial infections as it contains disinfecting properties, can also be used as an antilithic for bladder and kidney stones and cloudy urine; with Yerba Mansa and Slippery Elm, makes a great sitz bath herb for postpartum stitches and tears; will stimulate oxytocin. (NP)

Valerian *(Valeriana spp.)* Acts as a nerve tonic for irritations, hysteria, restlessness and emotional stress; good for pain and intestinal and menses cramps.

Virginia Snake Root *(Aristolochia serpentaria)* For constipation in a weak digestive tract and the elderly, it warms up the center of the body and stimulates metabolism, stimulates blood circulation in extremities and will increase appetite; also an immuno-stimulant to increase white blood cells. (NP)

White Oak *(Quercus alba)* This astringent herb is useful in gum inflammations, gingivitis, loose teeth and sore throats; also an intestinal tonic to diarrhea; due to high bioflavinoids, it can be used to strengthen capillary fragility for chronic nosebleeds, varicosities and hemorrhoids.

White Willow *(Salix alba)* Specifically due to salicin content, this herb will reduce inflammations of joints and membranes, finding use in headaches, fevers, arthritis and hay fever; useful in bladder infections acting as an analgesic to those tissues.

Wild Cherry *(Prunus virginiana)* Used for a hot, dry cough and mild bronchitis in children and adults, makes a good syrup; will resoften up bronchial mucus making it easier to expectorate and will keep lungs from drying out; soothing and cooling.

Wild Ginger *(Asarum canadensis)* For colds and viral infections to induce sweating; for crampy slow-starting menses; an immune potentiator. (NP)

Wild Sarsaparilla *(Aralia nudicaulis)* For anemia and low hematocrit, this plant is called a "coadaptogen" and will basically return an overactive or sluggish system to normalcy; considered an anabolic synergist, it acts to repair liver and kidney deficiency; has mild laxative effects and is a growth stimulant; works well with Licorice and Ginseng.

Wild Yam *(Dioscorea villosa)* Will soothe the nerves in neuralgia and pains of the urinary tract; also recommended for cramps; relieves pregnancy nausea and has use in threatened miscarriage.

Witch Hazel *(Hamamelis virginiana)* As a traditional remedy, used internally and as a liniment, it is applied to varicosities, varicose veins and hemorrhoids and any swollen engorged tissues; may help control diarrhea and ease dysentery in formulas.

Yarrow *(Achillea lanulosa)* Useful in colds, influenza, fevers and respiratory infections; dyspepsia and suppressed menses; will stop passive internal bleeding; coughing and spitting blood. (NP)

Yellow Dock *(Rumex crispus)* A blood purifier used for skin problems; contains easily digestible iron mineral; reduces accumulation of wastes; useful for rheumatism, ulcers, constipation and liver congestion from fatty foods; effective in skin eruptions related to menstrual cycle. (NP)

Yerba Mansa *(Anemopsis californica)* Good for rheumatoid arthritis, inflamed hemorrhoids, cystitis, appendicitis, bleeding gums and herpes lesions, hyperuricemia, preclampsia and the onset of allergies, very similar to Golden Seal in action and results.

Yerba Santa *(Eriodictyon californica)* Valuable for colds, chronic laryngitis, bronchitis, hay fever and asthma; leading agent for all respiratory problems; will dry up excess fluids in the lungs, being useful in excess mucous secretions.

Yohimbe *(Corynanthe)* For prostatitis associated with low self-esteem and low sperm count; for neurosis and stress causing decreased vasopressant; use in CONSERVATIVE amounts or can cause prostatitis. (NP)

Yucca *(Yucca glauca)* An anti-inflammatory for arthritic joints; allergy and auto-immune reactions causing hyaluronidase in the joints. (NP)

Herbal Combinations

ALLER AID *This formula is for hay fever symptoms of runny nose and watery eyes due to pollen and animal allergens yet will not create rebound symptoms like Ephedra or other antihistamines.*

Yerba Santa *(Eriodictyon californica)* traditionally used where there is an abundance of secretions, dries up and organizes the mucous membranes of the upper respiratory system.

Nettles *(Urtica gracilis)* being high in chlorophyll, helps the body produce natural antihistamines.

Eyebright *(Euphrasia officinalis)* acts as a tonic to tissues, strengthening the tensile structure of the eye, and reducing acrid eye and nose secretions.

Mormon Tea *(Ephedra torreyana)* has bronchio-dilating abilities, shrinks swollen tissues in the nose but without Ma Huang's side effects.

ATHLETES ENDURANCE *This combination increases physical endurance and stamina for peak performance levels, giving support to all body systems and increases vitamin absorption. (NP)*

Burdock *(Arctium minus)* decreases lactic acid in the joints and muscles, that reduces muscle soreness, and alkalinizes the blood helping to maintain electrolyte balances.

Oshá *(Ligusticum porteri)* increases bronchio-dilation to up oxygen intake and helps eliminate excess carbon dioxide build up in the blood, facilitating deeper breathing.

Gotu Kola *(Centella asiatica)* helps carry nutrients to the brain and enhances neural synaptic activity helping to rejuvenate the central nervous system.

Yerba Mansa *(Anemopsis californica)* protects cellular integrity, inhibiting inflammation, infection and tissue injury.

St. John's Wort *(Hypericum perforatum)* helps to lift the spirits when one is having the blues; is also anti-inflammatory and regenerative in nerve damage along the spinal cord.

American Ginseng *(Panax quinquefolium)* a premier adaptogen supports the body's ability to handle stresses.

Cayenne *(Capsicum spp.)* is an adjunct herb that helps carry the other herbs throughout the body and increases the body's ability to move blood to the extremities.

BITTER TONIC *For chronic stomach and intestinal problems, gas, heartburn and burping associated with digestive disorders, it can be taken 15 to 30 minutes before a heavy meal. It will stimulate digestive enzymes needed to break down and assimilate dietary fats and proteins.*

Gentian *(Swertia radiata)* increases blood supply to the stomach lining as well as HCL and pepsin production.

Cardamon *(Elettaria cardamomum)* is a spicy tonic to the upper GI where there is poor salivation and enzyme secretion.

Orange Peel is a carminative to relieve excess flatulence.

BREATHE DEEP *This combination has therapeutic value in colds, influenza, asthma, bronchitis, croup, emphysema, lung congestion and swollen glands. It facilitates the expectoration of mucus out of the bronchioles and contains Oshá, an herbal anti-viral useful in combating most flus. (NP)*

Oshá *(Ligusticum porteri)* is a bronchio dilator, antiviral to colds and flus, and an expectorant, that facilitates the upward movement of mucus out of the lungs.

Yerba Mansa *(Anemopsis californica)* an anti-microbial and anti-asthmatic, decreases inflammation and keeps the tissues free of bacterias.

Red Root *(Ceanothus fendleri)* drains the lymph, supports the immune system and helps it to clean up metabolic waste products.

Pleurisy *(Asclepias tuberosa)* is traditionally used for chronic infections characterized by hot, dry mucous membranes and dry skin with an inability to sweat.

Mullein *(Verbascum thapsus)* for where there is bronchiole irritability and spasming, is used here for its tonic and respiratory nerve relaxing properties to open the lungs.

BRIGHT EYES *This formula provides flavonoids that optimize vascular integrity of the eye, toning and strengthening the entire ocular stucture. The flavonoids relieve tired and weak eyes and aid in night and color blindness.*

Eyebright *(Eucalyptus golbulus)* is beneficial in acute and chronic eye inflammations, chronic tearing and over-sensitivity to light.

Blueberry *(Vaccimium myrtillus)* this shrubby plant regenerates impulses from the retina to the brain, fortifying visual purple, it may also guard against glaucoma.

Hawthorne *(caecrataegus succulenta)* it is a nutritive to the cardiovasuclar system including the arteriole endings in the eye, a tonic to connective tissue and lowers high blood pressure.

Ginkgo (Ginkgo biloba) the flavons in this plant dilate cerebral blood vessels, enhancing blood flow and oxygen to the head.

CALM A KID *This combination relaxes, sedates and nourishes the nervous system; stops internal chatter and hyper states in children or adults; promotes a restful sleep and is an excellent remedy for keeping sick children restful.*

Hops *(Humulus lupulus)* is useful for insomnia and hyperkinetic conditions in kids.

Catnip *(Nepeta cataria)* relieves agitation, nervousness or anxiety.

Skullcap *(Scutellaria lateriflora)* a restorative tonic, helps to take the edge off excess pain and relieve discomfort.

Passion Flower *(Passiflora incarnata)* is useful in nervous insomnia and sadness.

Oat Seed *(Avena fatua/sativa)* a neural nourisher, has abilities to rebuild and restore the nervous system.

Pulsatilla *(Pulsatilla patens)* is used in highly agitated emotional states with gloom and distress.

Black Cohosh *(Cimicifuga racemosa)* helps relieve dull aching, headaches or extremity pains.

CANDA-TONIC *This combination inhibits candida reproduction in the intestinal tract; useful in all systemic yeast infections; will also help support the immune system.*

Pau D'Arco *(Tabebuia impeteginosa)* inhibits candida's ability to reproduce.

Desert Willow *(Chilopsis linearis)* with action that is identical to Pau D'Arco, is a local U.S. plant, making it more ecological to use.

Usnea *(Usnea spp.)* inhibits excess yeast infections without effecting healthy flora in the GI tract.

Echinacea *(Echinacea angustifolia)* increases white blood cell production and activates the immune response.

Yerba Mansa *(Anemopsis californica)* prevents the breakdown of the gastrointestinal lining caused by flora imbalances.

Chaparro Amargosa *(Castela emoryi)* inhibits intestinal protozoa and candida overgrowth.

Dandelion *(Taraxacum officinale)* relieves excess fluid imbalances in the GI tract created by candida inflammation.

CATNIP-FENNEL FORMULA *This simple remedy is for indigestion from improper food combinations and over eating; with gas and hiccoughs. Makes a pleasant after dinner tea if added to a cup of hot water.*

Catnip *(Nepeta cataria)* relieves intestinal cramping and pain.

Fennel *(Foeniculum spp.)* provides antispasmodic actions to "double over" cramping.

Peppermint *(Mentha piperita)* besides adding a pleasant minty taste to this combination, relaxes nervous spasms in the stomach.

CIRCULA-FLOW *This combination is used to strengthen the heart muscle and regulate heart beat as well as helping to remove plaque along the arterial wall.*

Hawthorne *(Crataegus succulenta)* a premier cardiac tonic, strengthens the heart muscle.

Yarrow *(Achillea lanulosa)* prevents internal hemorrhaging and strengthens the whole cardiovascular system.

Kelp *(Nereocystis luetkeana)* provides valuable nutrients and minerals that help the blood keep its charge.

Garlic *(Allium sativa)* lowers high cholesterol that leads to high blood pressure.

Cayenne *(Capsicum spp.)* redistributes blood throughout the body, relieving pressure on the heart.

CLEAR SKIN *This liver and blood cleansing combination is used for acne, abscesses, eczema, psoriasis, scalp irritations, rashes, insect bites and most skin eruptions by stimulating the liver to increase blood filtration and maintain proper blood pH balances. It is also useful in most chronic constipation problems. (NP)*

Echinacea *(Echinacea angustifolia)* stimulates the immune system's ability to help clean up the blood.

Burdock *(Arctium minus)* resupplies the skin with natural oils while keeping acne at bay.

Yellow Dock *(Rumex crispus)* decongests the liver by stimulating bile production, helping with dietary fat absorption.

Oregon Grape *(Mahonia repens)* is useful in food and skin allergies by increasing the body's ability to digest proteins.

Yarrow *(Achillea lanulosa)* opens the pores of the skin to increase elimination of metabolic wastes.

Wild Sarsaparilla *(Aralia nudicaulis)* repairs liver deficiency with mild laxative effects and increases red blood cell count.

CREATIVITY *These herbs increase arterial circulation to the head therefore enhancing memory recall and the capacity to concentrate. Ginkgo is also known to have positive benefits in Alzheimer's disease. (NP)*

Ginkgo *(Ginkgo biloba)* increases mental alertness and aptitude by increasing cerebral blood supply and oxygen.

Gotu Kola *(Centella asiatica)* increases neural synapses and carries nutrients through the nervous system, rejuvenating brain cells, giving food for thought.

Rosemary *(Rosmarinus officinalis)* "The Herb of Remembrance", it enhances dreams and gives an invigorating scent to the brain, normalizing low blood pressure and strengthening capillaries in the head.

American Ginseng *(Panax quinquefolium)* as an adaptogen, increases nerve fiber growth and prevents nerve damage from radiation and decreases blood cholesterol.

Virginia Snake Root *(Aristolochia serpentaria)* increases visceral and peripheral circulation, enhancing abilities of the other herbs.

ECHINACEA ADVANTAGE *This combination enhances Echinacea's ability to travel through the system and deliver it's immune boosting action.*

Echinacea *(Echinacea angustifolia/purpurea)* using the whole plant gives a full array of constituents, prevents the breakdown and inflammation of injured tissues from allergies to colds and flus.

Spearmint *(Mentha spicata)* furthers the action and imparts a pleasant taste, making the formula more effective.

Prickly Ash *(Xanthoxylum americanum)* increases nervous and circulatory system action, toning and cleansing the stomach and increasing blood supply to all visceral organs.

ECHINACEA - GOLDEN SEAL *This energetic combination is effective in cleaning up any illness that secretes toxins into the blood. As an antibacterial, it stimulates the healing process by increasing the white blood cell count to the area of infection, relieving colds, flus, sores, infections and bacterial and viral eruptions internally or externally. (NP)*

Echinacea *(Echinacea angustifolia)* turns on the immune system to fight acute, infectious stages of disease.

Golden Seal *(Hydrastis canadensis)* a powerful herbal antibiotic, it stimulates removal of thick and tenacious mucus secretions that have a tendency to ulcerate the membranes in infections.

ECHINACEA - OSHÁ RECIPE *This formula is excellent for upper respiratory infections and the first sign of colds, flus and fevers; it soothes a sore throat, thins bronchial mucus; is antibacterial, anti-viral and mucolitic. (NP)*

Echinacea *(Echinacea angustifolia)* keeps the immune system functioning at its peak, draining the lymph.

Oshá *(Ligusticum porteri)* a powerful anti-viral, soothes sore throats and facilitates the removal of excess mucus in the bronchioles.

Inmortal *(Asclepias asperula)* increases secretions to dry sinuses and lungs where mucus is stuck making it hard to breathe or cough anything up.

Licorice *(Glycyrrhiza glabra)* a mucolytic, dilutes thick mucus making it easier to eliminate and imparts a pleasant taste that harmonizes this recipe.

ELDER'S HERBAL *This combination stimulates blood circulation toning the whole cardiovascular system and strengthening the liver. It improves cellular function to the brain enhancing memory and mental alertness.*

Ginkgo *(Ginkgo biloba)* for arteriosclerotic symptoms with minimal cerebral blood supply, does not mix with serious prescriptions.

Hawthorne *(Crataegus succulenta)* useful in hypertension and myocardial weaknesses, does not mix with beta blockers.

Milk Thistle *(Silybum marianum)* protects liver cells from damage that may be caused by radiation, alcohol, solvents and chemicals.

American Ginseng *(Panax quinquefolium)* helps to reduce high blood sugar and elevated uric acid, helping the body defeat long term stress.

Virginia Snake Root *(Aristolochia serpentaria)* increases absorption of vitamins A, D and E and dietary fats.

Gotu Kola *(Centella asiatica)* useful in sluggish metabolism with mild hypothyroid levels, increases oxygen and nutrients to the head, allowing one to think more clearly.

Nettles *(Urtica gracilis)* high in chlorophyll, gives nutritional supplementation.

Cayenne *(Capsicum spp.)* acts as a synergist to carry the other herbs through the system.

ELEMENT SUPPLEMENT *This combination replaces minerals in the body depleted by everyday stress. Contains iron, calcium, iodine, potassium, phosphorus and silica. As free mineral ions, it replaces loss of electrolytes.*

Alfalfa *(Medicago sativa)* alkalinizes the pH and proteins in the blood, a recuperative herb that increases assimilation of all nutrients.

Kelp *(Nereocystis luetkeana)* a sea veggie with high calcium content, is known as a radiation antagonist.

Yellow Dock *(Rumex crispus)* releases stored iron in the liver and increases assimilation of dietary fats.

Nettles *(Urtica gracilis)* high in chlorophyll, iron and calcium, makes it a premier blood builder.

Wild Sarsaparilla *(Aralia nudicaulis)* is a blood tonic and immunological strengthener.

Horsetail *(Equisetum arvense)* with a high silica content, gives this herb collagen astringency and tonic effects for connective tissue weaknesses.

FEVERFEW-CLEMATIS COMPOUND *For headaches from constipation, alcohol or sinus infections, this formula will decrease spasms and vascular pooling to and from the brain. Migraines may be helped. (NP)*

Feverfew *(Chrysanthemum parthenium)* an anti-inflammatory, relieves headaches, migraines and PMS.

Clematis *(Clematis spp.)* relieves frontal and migraine headaches with a sweaty neck and fore head that doesn't respond to OTC drugs.

Black Cohosh *(Cimicifuga racemosa)* alleviates headaches around the eyes and forehead and dull aches in the muscles.

Skullcap *(Scutellaria lateriflora)* eases head pain that may originate from spinal cord injuries or misalignments.

GINSENG FLING *This ginseng combination is a premier constitutional tonic with adaptogenic properties giving the body an improved ability to adapt to the stresses of life. (NP).*

Woodsgrown American Ginseng *(Panax quinquefolium)* decreases stress effects from bad habits and leaking away of energy, improving blood circulation with an anti-aging factor that increases strength and stamina.

Wild American Ginseng leaf *(Panax quinquefolium)* using only the leaf, preserves this dwindling species' roots for future yearly growth yet imparts the potency of the wild plant.

Siberian Ginseng *(Eleutherococcus senticosis)* is used for long standing anabolic stress that may result in depression, anorexia or neurasthenia where the adrenals and the nervous system are shot.

Spikenard root & berry *(Aralia racemosa)* similar to ginseng in action, buffers stress references in the brain.

Licorice *(Glycyrrhiza glabra)* supports exhausted adrenals with poor gastro-intestinal function, constipation or an ulcerous system.

Motherwort *(Leonurus cardiaca)* for stress induced hypertension, relaxes the blood vessels, and grounds a person out.

Oat Seed *(Avena sativa)* a rich neural nourisher, aids nervous exhaustion.

GINSENG-LICORICE FORMULA *These adaptogenic herbs help to support and nourish the adrenals by increasing constitutional vitality and endurance and helping the body deal with various stresses. (NP).*

American Ginseng *(Panax quinquefolium)* is excellent for stress induced wasting diseases.

Devil's Claw *(Harpagophytum procumbens)* as an anti-inflammatory, supports the adrenal cortex and lowers the amount of hormones needed to run daily maintenance.

Licorice *(Glycyrrhiza glabra/lepidota)* helps increase the efficiency and recyclability of adrenal hormones without taxing the adrenals.

GUARANA KOLA NUT COMPOUND *This reviving formula will increase circulation and boost the adrenals without the allergens found in coffee. It does contain caffeine.*

Guarana *(Paullinia cupana)* is useful in weight reduction programs, hangovers and headaches.

Kola Nut *(Cola nitida)* supplies blood to the skeletal muscles and is mildly hypertensive.

Damiana *(Turnera diffusa)* helps nervous depression with poor appetite.

Virginia Snake Root *(Aristolochia serpentaria)* is a blood and nervous system stimulant.

GUM TONER *Promoting healthy gums and mouth, this combination is good for pyorrhea, gingivitis, sore throats, swollen lymph nodes and strep throat where it is difficult to swallow. It can be used as a gargle and should be swallowed.*

Propolis *(Propolis)* a topical anti-septic and analgesic, shortens healing time for any skin, mouth or throat soreness.

Myrrh Gum *(Commiphora molmol)* useful for pharyngitis, stimulates immune response to infections.

Spearmint *(Mentha spicata)* imparts a pleasant taste to bitter herbs and deodorizes the breath.

ITCH AWAY *These herbs are soothing and helpful in poison oak and ivy inflammations and skin rashes as a liniment.*

Grindelia *(Grindelia squarrosa)* forms a lacquer coating on the skin, cools and prevents spreading from itching.

Plantain *(Plantago major)* soothing and anti-inflammatory to the skin, promotes healing.

Witch Hazel *(Hamamelis virginiana)* helps drying and is astringent.

IMMUNE SUPPORT *Allergies, daily stress and autoimmune diseases constantly tax the immune system's capacity. These tonic herbs deeply replenish a compromised system and can act pro-phylacticaly as a preventative to immune malfunction.*

Astragalus *(Astragalus membranicus)* this herb is traditionally used in Chinese medicine for chronic and persistent infections and wasting diseases by achieving complete immune restoration.

Reishi *(Ganoderma lucidum)* this woody mushroom is shown to assist the immune system to prevent tumors and attack malignant cells while stimulating the body's own defenses.

Cat's Claw *(Uncaria tomensosa)* this Peruvian vine is shown to decrease fatigue in chemically sensitive individuals, relieving depression and enhancing immune function.

Red Root *(Ceanothus fendleri)* a long term tonic, it shrinks non-fibrous cysts by stimulating lymphatic circulation and drainage. Good for people with high fat diets, it increases osmolity, by making the blood have a better electrical charge, lowering density lipids.

Burdock root *(Arctium minus)* eliminates excess metabolic waste products in the blood from low level toxicity and aids liver congestion by pulling out poisons in the system.

Siberian Gingeng *(Eleutherococcus senticosis)* being an adaptogen, it supports longevity and endurance levels.

Cleavers *(Galium)* clinical studies show the fluid extract suspends cancerous ulcers and is traditionally used for lymphatic swelling with gentle, soothing action.

KID'S FOCUS POWER *This formula is for children with learning disabilities and a diminished ability to concentrate, control impulses and screen out irrelevant stimuli. Once diet and nutrient deficiencies are considered, these herbs have shown beneficial calming and restorative action on the brain and nervous system. They have shown to relax children with chronic anxiety.*

Green Tea *(Camellia sinensia)* traditionally in other cultures, hyperactive children are given a cup of coffee a day for caffeine, to slow down and enhance their ability to focus. This herb has similar yet milder caffeine levels without all the allergenic oils of coffee and has the added benefit of bioflavanoids.

Motherwort *(Leonurus cardiaca)* a very useful plant in an overexcited nervous system where sensory and motor functions are all out of proportion. It grounds out the individual and relaxes the circulatory system, easing heart palpitations.

Passion Flower *(Passiflora incarnata)* this plant elevates the mood, relieving depression that may accompany nervous irritability. Calms and normalizes the cardiovascular system.

Oat Seed *(Avena sativa/fatua)* a nerual nourisher, the milky juice of this seed revitalizes and strenghtens the nervous system; it controls nervous exhaustion and decreases anxiety and fragile emotional states.

Lemon Balm *(Melissa officianalis)* this aromatic plant corrects insomnia and disturbed sleep patterns facilitating a more restful deep sleep and has a relaxed overall influence without causing drowsiness.

LIFT THE SPIRITS HERBAL ADVANTAGE *For those who experience "the blues", sadness from depression, produces a feeling of well being and increasing sociability, oxygenizing the brain to think clearer and nourishing the nervous system.*

Kava Kava *(Piper methysticum)* a non-addicting euphoretic, aids in relaxing the body yet increases communicativeness and informality.

St. John's Wort *(Hypericum perforatum)* helps with agitation, depression, nervous exhaustion and anxiety, a remedy for the general grouchies.

Passion Flower *(Passiflora incarnata)* functions as a mood elevator, enhancing circulation with toning effects to the sympathetic nerve centers.

Ginkgo *(Ginkgo biloba)* useful in impaired cerebral blood supply, returns elasticity to major arteries.

Kelp *(Nereocystis luetkeana)* is an excellent mineral replacer for nervous system nutrients.

Lavender *(Lavendula officinalis)* increases cerebral blood flow through its beneficial scent.

Oat Seed *(Avena sativa/fatua)* is a deep neural tonic and restorative.

American Ginseng *(Panax quinquefolium)* a premier adaptogen, supports stress induced nervous system disorders.

Lemon *(Citrus limon)* a refreshing flavor to this combination, imparts a cool, harmonizing taste.

LIMBER UP *This combination may increase joint mobility and expand the range of motion for sore, stiff joints and muscles; arthritis, gout, rheumatism and bursitis. It decreases urea and lactic acid deposits from metabolic waste due to inflammations and will therefore decrease the inflammation.* (NP)

Devil's Claw *(Harpagophytum procumbens)* a prostaglandin inhibitor to the joints, supports the adrenals.

Yucca *(Yucca glauca)* with cortisone-like properties, relieves pain in the joints by breaking down organic wastes like uric acid.

Yerba Mansa *(Anemopsis californica)* for slow healing conditions, supports the immune system, stimulates fluid transport in boggy, swollen joints and prevents the further breakdown of cartilage.

Burdock seed *(Arctium minus)* a natural diuretic, useful in all allergic type reactions, keeps the blood clean.

Alfalfa *(Medicago sativa)* alkalinizes an acid ridden blood stream and replaces lost nutrients.

Yarrow *(Achillea lanulosa)* returns tone to swollen tissues and increases digestive efficiency.

Cayenne *(Capsicum spp.)* increases peripheral vasodilation and blood transport, helping to clean up retrograde metabolism.

LMPH FLOW *Used for tonsillitis, swollen glands, enlarged spleen, lymphatic congestion, infections and inflammations, it stimulates the immune response by supporting the lymphatic system.* (NP)

Red Root *(Ceanothus fendleri)* supports the structural aspects of the lymphatic circulatory system and shrinks cysts and tumors by increasing the drainage of swollen tissues.

Burdock *(Arctium minus)* deacidifies the blood, alkalinizing the pH and supports the liver to cleanse the body relieving waste products from inflammations.

Echinacea *(Echinacea angustifolia)* as an antibacterial, stimulates white blood cells to an area of infection, reduces tissue dissolution and speeds up a slow healing process.

Yerba Mansa *(Anemopsis californica)* as a hyaluronidase inhibitor, decreases inflammation and reduces tissue damage in injured cells.

Ocotillo *(Fouqueria splendens)* specifically drains the lymph in the pelvis finding use in intestinal infections.

Stillingia *(Stillingia sylvatica)* is a lymphatic drainer to the respiratory system with a slow recuperative process.

Blue Flag *(Iris missouriensis)* a powerful liver lymphatic, increases the body's metabolism.

LVR HARMONICS *For poor digestion aggravated by fats, alcohol or coffee; it helps with hangovers and dullness in the morning. This beneficial formula is useful for painters, stain glass workers, mechanics or anyone working around industrial solvents or environmental pollutants. (NP)*

Echinacea *(Echinacea angustifolia)* stimulates the blood cleansing abilities of the immune system, and controls septic conditions that liver congestion can cause.

Barberry *(Berberis fendleri)* increases the liver's ability to breakdown hydrocarbons and other toxins that otherwise get stored here.

Toadflax *(Linaria vulgaris)* is specific for tiredness that's associated with liver backlog of catabolic wastes; specific for hangover symptoms whatever the cause.

Fringetree *(Chionanthus virginicus)* relieves dull liver pain due to bile blockage; nausea in the morning and light colored stools.

Dandelion *(Taraxacum officinale)* a liver cooler and blood alkalinizer, helps dilate the portal artery, increasing blood circulation through the liver.

Blue Flag *(Iris missouriensis)* aids individuals with a poor over-processed diet or the inability to digest food well.

MALE VITALITY *This combination increases male virility by toning the reproductive organs and strengthening prostate function and testosterone levels. Some of the herbs in this formula seem to enhance sexual responses by increasing sensitivity. (NP)*

Dong Quai *(Angelica sinensis)* increases steroidal binding sites to testosterone sensitive cells, for prostatic and testicular deficiencies, helping balance the hormones.

Saw Palmetto *(Serenoa serrulata)* a prostate tonic, helps nourish the tissues of the male reproductive system; useful in dribbling, dull ache and no rectal problems.

American Ginseng *(Panax quinquefolium)* finds service in stress induced hormonal imbalances and uric acid elevation.

Wild Sarsaparilla *(Aralia nudicaulis)* is specific for benign prostatic hypertrophy with poor immunologic strength and deficient steroid production.

Dandelion *(Taraxacum officinale)* helps the anabolic stressed individual with sodium retention high blood pressure.

Virginia Snake Root *(Aristolochia serpentaria)* for malabsorption of dietary oils and vitamins in poor lipid metabolism, moves the blood and increases circulation in the nerves.

MELLOW OUT *This combination relaxes, calms and tones the nerves; it has antispasmodic properties to muscles and organs; it is good for insomnia, general neuralgia, anxiety and muscular twitching. (NP)*

Skullcap *(Scutellaria lateriflora)* lessens surface irritability to acupuncture, massage, spinal adjustments; traditionally used in nocturnal seizures.

Passion Flower *(Passiflora incarnata)* as a muscle relaxant and arterial sedative, shows service in nervous insomnia and lifts the spirits.

Hops *(Humulus lupulus)* for nervous stomach and colon spasms, relaxes hyperkinetic conditions.

St. John's Wort *(Hypericum perforatum)* for stress induced agitation and depression, a remedy for the blues.

American Ginseng *(Panax quinquefolium)* helps with stress that sets off limbic system hyperfunctions; it gives back the subjective sense of well being.

MENO VITAPAUSE *This promotes a smooth transition by easing menopausal changes. It supports the adrenals, helps with constipation, dry skin, vaginal dryness (along with a Calendula/St. John's Wort oil lubricant) and mood swings. (NP)*

> **Dong Quai** (*Angelica sinensis*) increases the available uptake of estrogen the body still makes thus increasing the nourishment of reproductive cells.
>
> **Dandelion** (*Taraxacum officinale*) minimizes bloating, weight gain and cerebral edema that leads to irritability and mood swings.
>
> **Licorice** (*Glycyrrhiza glabra*) moisturizes the mucous membranes, mimicking estrogen's response in the body.
>
> **Motherwort** (*Leonurus cardiaca*) as a cardiovascular tonic, helps with hot flashes and heart palpitations from stress and allows one to feel more grounded and less volatile.
>
> **Hawthorne** (*Crataegus succulenta*) strengthens the heart and eases stress related hypertension and myocardial weaknesses.
>
> **Burdock** (*Arctium minus*) a uterine tonic and strengthener, helps to keep the blood clean and increases the liver's circulatory abilities.
>
> **Cayenne** (*Capsicum spp.*) helps to increase motility of the other herbs, increases the circulation to the skin and mucous membranes for dry skin and vagina.

MENSES HELPER *Used for chronic menses pain, discharge, excessive bleeding and irregular periods. It will tone the reproductive organs and help regulate periods to be on time. (NP)*

> **Aletris** (*Aletris farinosa*) relieves constipation and gas that accompanies the menses cycle.
>
> **Partridge Berry** (Squaw Vine) (*Mitchella repens*) a uterine tonic, supports the whole reproductive system and quiets nervous irritability and reduces bloating.
>
> **Blue Cohosh** (*Caulophyllum thalictroides*) is specific for heavy bearing down sensation that goes with crampy or slow starting cycle.
>
> **Cramp Bark** (*Viburnum opulus*) alleviates referred pain that runs through the sacral and leg area; a muscle and neural relaxant.

MILK THISTLE COMPOUND *This Chaparral alternative acts to leach heavy metals and radiation toxicity from the thyroid, blood and liver as well as protects the liver against further damage. (NP)*

> **Milk Thistle** (*Silybum marianum*) supports one rehabilitating from alcohol or long term solvent exposure, reducing fatty degeneration of liver cells and overt damage from chemicals.
>
> **Burdock** (*Arctium minus*) reduces allergic type reactions due to elevated uric acid in the blood.
>
> **Kelp** (*Nereocystis luetkeana*) as an electrolyte supporter and radiation antagonist, helps decongest the thyroid.
>
> **Blue Flag** (*Iris missouriensis*) supports a sluggish, congested liver with constipation or chronic tiredness with a backlog of harmful chemicals stored in the liver; stimulates immune function.

NURSING MOTHER'S SUPPORT *Used to stimulate lactation and increase quality of breast milk, these herbs are high in minerals especially calcium and magnesium.*

> **Fennel** (*Foeniculum vulgare*) helps with infant colic if taken 15 minutes before nursing to allow sufficient time to enter breast milk.
>
> **Blessed Thistle** (*Cnicus benedictus*) relieves baby or mother when they have loose stools due to metabolism being off and the rhythm hasn't been established yet.
>
> **Raspberry** (*Rubus idaeus*) cuts down on post partum bleeding, retones the uterus and increases calcium content to enrich the colostrum.
>
> **Burdock** (*Arctium minus*) through the milk, helps alleviate baby's skin rashes, retones mom's reproductive system and keeps the blood clean.

Red Clover (*Trifolium pratense*) as a nutritive, it is high in minerals, antispasmodic to respiratory problems and calming and soothing to babies.

NATURAL RESISTANCE *This combination stimulates the immune system; has anti-bacterial action; is excellent for colds, flus and infections. (NP-with discretion)*

Echinacea (Echinacea angustifolia) stimulates innate or surface immunity to help minimize allergic reactions and increase white blood cell production at the area of infection.

Pau D' Arco (Tabebuia impeteginosa) traditionally used in South America to successfully treat cancer and other auto immune diseases by fortifying the immune system.

Usnea (*Usnea spp.*) is an herbal antibiotic similar to penicillin but without causing yeast over growth in the G.I. tract.

Golden Seal (*Hydrastis canadensis*) a mucous membrane stimulator, tones the gastro-intestinal tract and lungs with highly anti-bacterial properties.

Propolis (*Propolis*) a tonic, aids damaged tissues from infections like strep throat and tonsillitis.

Wild Ginger (*Asarum canadensis*) an immune potentiator, helps break up a cold, warming the body to aid in sweating.

Cayenne (*Capsicum spp.*) facilitates delivery of the other herbs to the farthest reaches of the body and promotes sweating to eliminate toxins from illness.

NATURAL RESISTANCE FOR KIDS *Slightly syrupy in consistency, this combination is not only effective but tastes good too. Excellent for colds, flus and infections. Does not contain honey; safe for children under the age of one. Best for kids up to 5 or 6 years old.*

Echinacea (*Echinacea angustifolia*) stimulates immediate immune response for all illnesses and diseases, loosens stuck mucous in the lungs; facilitating better expectoration.

Burdock (*Arctium minus*) helps keep the blood from getting too acidic with metabolic wastes from illness by-products and helpful with sick headaches.

Pansy (*Viola tricolor*) helps for feverish conditions; a child's herbal aspirin.

Yarrow (*Achillea lanulosa*) opens the pores of the skin so toxins can be eliminated and helps to bring the fever down naturally.

Red Clover (*Trifolium pratense*) relieves coughs and hyperactivity allowing the child to relax and promotes a better quality sleep.

Lemon Thyme (*Thymus citrodorus*) a pleasant tasting herb, gently enhances the immune system and calms irritability.

Marshmallow (*Althea officinalis*) stimulates the immune system to increase white blood cells to fight invading pathogens, bacterias and toxins. It quells a sore throat and protects the mucous membranes from further invasions such as air borne viruses.

NAUSEA CALM *This formula is used for morning sickness, motion sickness and general nausea, and should be mixed in apple juice or a sweetened drink.*

Wild Yam (*Dioscorea villosa*) a prostaglandin inhibitor and stomach antispasmodic, quells cramps and relieves sudden nauseousness.

Cramp Bark (*Viburnum opulus*) useful for obstinate hiccoughs relaxing the diaphragm and stomach contractions.

Wild Ginger (*Asarum canadensis*) an antispasmodic that warms the stomach.

Peppermint (*Mentha piperita*) useful for difficult digestion and helps to mask the taste of bitter herbs.

PRE-MENSEASE *These herbs are good for premenstrual syndrome and irregular periods. It will help to balance estrogen/progesterone levels. (NP)*

ChasteTree (*Vitex agnus-castus*) Is useful for menses cycles longer than 28 days or progesterone deficiency syndromes like PMS. As a normalizer, it may help to shrink estrogen-dependent fibroids.

Black Haw (*Viburnum prunifolium*) reduces clotting an[...]
back pain in menses where the cramps may be rhythmic [...]

Raspberry (*Rubus idaeus*) a long term tonic and nourish[...]
ChasteTree berry.

Dandelion (*Taraxacum officinale*) reduces excess weight g[...]
accompanies PMS.

REJUVENATION
*This combination will promote longevity, induc[...]
system. It can be used for sluggish, chronic conditions and long[...]*

Astragalus (*Astragalus membranaceus*) as a deep immune t[...]
resistance to any illnesses and can be used in chronic and aut[...]
term benefits.

Gotu Kola (*Centella asiatica*) for conditions that depress thyr[...]
metabolism making one sluggish in all body functions, stimulat[...]

Virginia Snake Root (*Aristolochia serpentaria*) increases poor [...]
suppressed sweating and hot, dry skin with possible constipation[...]

Nettles (*Urtica gracilis*) act as an alkalinizing diuretic and miner[...]
phyll with natural antihistamine properties finding usefulness in a[...]

American Ginseng (*Panax quinquefolium*) as an adaptogen, it is l[...]
going to the source at the limbic system in the brain to cut down o[...]
body and supports the adrenals' overall function.

Cayenne (*Capsicum spp.*) facilitates blood movement and herbal d[...]
herbs do their job better.

ROMANTIC VIRTUE
*This formula will stimulate and tone up reproductiv[...]
romantic desires. It increases neural synapses and cuts down on emotio[...]
hinder the sensual flow. (NP)*

American Ginseng (*Panax quinquefolium*) decreases stress interferenc[...]
emotional sense of well being; enhances performance, increasing endur[...]

Gotu Kola (*Centella asiatica*) increases neural synapses giving new patl[...]
and improving response levels.

Damiana (*Turnera diffusa*) increases sex drive; useful for constant anxie[...]
about sexual matters, fear of no arousal, lubrication or erection.

Saw Palmetto (*Serenoa serrulata*) increases libido as a male and female r[...]

Passion Flower (*Passiflora incarnata*) acts as an appropriate mood elevato[...]
relaxant.

Cardamom (*Elettaria cardamomum*) as a carminative, inhibits any digestiv[...]

SLEEP EASY
*For restless and nervous insomnia. It will help with the individua[...]
at 3 a.m. still processing daily matters. It helps one to fall asleep faster and sleep[...]*

Valerian (*Valeriana spp.*) increases the quality of deep sleep and reduces the [...]
taken to fall asleep; a premier nervous system relaxant for insomnia and pain i[...]
irritability, specifically those with a sluggish constitutional nature.

Hops (*Humulus lupulus*) alleviates muscle spasms and leg cramps that keep on[...]
into a deep sleep.

Skullcap (*Scutellaria lateriflora*) reduces hyperfunctions and nocturnal neuropa[...]
evening hyperkinetic individual; also takes the edge off of any type of pain from s[...]
myalgia.

THROAT SPRAY
more area thar[...]
and are benefi[...]
antiviral agent[...]

Oshá (*Li[...]
Usnea (l[...]
to white[...]
Licorice[...]
tissues;[...]
Echina[...]
like str[...]

URISOOTHE[...]
bladder an[...]

Marsh[...]
memb[...]
Asper[...]
and i[...]
Yerba[...]
to ba[...]
Pips[...]
muc[...]
Cor[...]
fron[...]
as a[...]
Ho[...]
spa[...]

URITON[...]
functio[...]

P[...]
a[...]
a[...]

J[...]
h[...]

r[...]

When extracts are misted onto the mucous membranes of the throat, they cover
when simply swallowed. The herbs in this formula will quell a dry, hacking cough
ial to where it hurts to swallow. Acting as an anti-inflammatory, anitbacterial and
this spray soothes and re-moistens hot, dry and inflamed mucous membranes.

usticum porteri) upper respiratory antiviral and anesthetic to a sore throat.

snea spp.) highly antibiotic having similarities to penicillin and immuno-stimulating
blood cells.

(*Glycyrrhiza glabra*) a re-moistening agent that produces a protective coating on the
also anti-inflammatory with cortisone-like properties.

ea (*Echinacea angustifolia*) anti-viral, anti-bacterial on certain gram-positive bacteria
p and staph, also immuno-stimulating with interferon action.

*For hot, active infections of the urinary tract, it will soothe and cool out kidney,
urethra inflammations.*

nallow (*Althea officinalis*) an immune stimulant, forms a protective coating on mucus
ranes of the bladder and urethra, soothing out hot inflammations and absorbing toxins.

(*Populus tremuloides*) high in salicilates, functions similar to aspirin with fever, pain
flammation reducing properties.

Mansa (*Anemopsis californica*) lowers acid levels in urine from infection, antimicrobial
terial or viral infections, helps to minimize damage to injured and swollen tissues.

ssewa (*Chimaphila umbellata*) is specific for difficult urination with little urine but with
us and strong odor.

Silk (*Zea mays*) increases the volume of urine and therefore dilute any solid wastes
infectious by-products; traditionally used in chronic bladder infections, even in children,
urinary sedative.

setail (*Equisetum arvense*) relieves irritation due to the presence of urinary calculi and
smic urging to urinate, particularly at night, in acute inflammations.

*For sluggish, chronic, low grade urinary infections; tones up and stimulates organ
ing.*

sissewa (*Chimaphila umbellata*) is used in chronic conditions with mucous, scanty urine
d cloudy urate dust; specific for chronic low grade kidney infections related to arthritis or
to immune type syndromes.

niper Berry (*Juniperus communis*) for weak kidneys without an active inflammation;
ings heat and tones the urinary system.

yrrh Gum (*Commiphora molmol*) returns tone to any mucus membrane that is chronically
cerated due to long standing inflammations, increases red blood cells and activates the
mmune response.

Agrimony (*Agrimonia eupatoria*) useful in cloudy, smelly urine and cystorrhea, helps
alkalinize an acid urine.

Corn Silk (*Zea mays*) for chronic pain in cystitis or urethritis; an astringent to the mucus
membranes, pulling out excess mucous and helpful in incontinence.

SYRUPS

HOREHOUND - MARSHMALLOW SYRUP *This syrup is slightly milder than the Oshá-Wild Cherry Syrup but still contains Oshá in the formula. It is indicated for children and adults with the kind of loose rattling cough that just needs a little support to facilitate. The Horehound relaxes the lungs and reduces feverish symptoms while the Marshmallow soothes and coats the throat.*

Horehound (*Marrubium vulgare*), Oshá (*Ligusticum porteri*), Marshmallow (*Althea officinalis*) Honey, Brandy, Lime

OSHÁ-WILD CHERRY SYRUP *This syrup is best for hot, dry, feverish conditions with little or no expectoration but plenty of congestion and hot sore throat. Oshá is anti-viral and anti-bacterial making it excellent for sinus and upper respiratory infections, colds and flus.*

Oshá (*Ligusticum porteri*), Wild Cherry (*Prunus virginiana*), White Pine (*Pinus strobus*), Spikenard (*Aralia racemosa*), Poplar (*Populus sargentii*), Bloodroot (*Sanguinaria canadensis*), honey, vodka, almond extract, vegetable glycerine

MARSHMALLOW KIDS SYRUP *This syrup is especially designed for children under two years and anyone who cannot tolerate honey. It is sweetened with barley malt and maple syrup. The Marshmallow coats and protects the mucus membranes of the throat and bronchioles. This syrup is indicated for anyone needing anti-microbial action.*

Horehound (*Marrabium vulgare*), Echinacea (*Echinacea angustifolia*), Marshmallow (*Althea officinalis*), Oshá (*Ligusticum porteri*), barley malt, maple syrup, brandy, almond extract, vegetable glycerine

SALVES

CALENDULA-COMFREY SKIN DRESSING *This salve prevents scarring, speeds up healing of burns, sun or wind, good for pregnancy stretch marks and during lactation. Good for herpes and healing surgical stitches.*

Calendula Flowers (*Calendula officinalis*), Comfrey Root and Leaf (*Symphytum officinale*), Almond Oil, Olive Oil, Beeswax, Vitamin E

SHOTGUN SKIN DRESSING *This salve is used for sunburn, diaper rash, hemorrhoids, herpes lesions, abrasions, swellings, insect bites, infections. Anti-microbial, emollient and astringent. It gets results quickly.*

Comfrey (*Symphytum officinale*), Marshmallow (*Althea officinalis*), Golden Seal (*Hydrastis canadensis*), Bloodroot (*Sanguinaria canadensis*), Chaparral (*Larrea glutinosa*), Yerba Mansa (*Anemopsis californica*), Oshá (*Ligusticum porteri*), Bistort (*Polygonum bistorta*), Myrrh gum (*Commiphora molmol*), Echinacea (*Echinacea angustifolia*), Almond Oil, Safflower Oil, Beeswax

CORDIALS

DANDELION CORDIAL *A pleasant tasting cordial for the individual with an over acidic constitution that tends towards ulcers, arteriosclerosis and gallstones; helps with digestion of fats and proteins, decreases uric acid concentrations and water retention and elevated blood fats.*

Dandelion (*Taraxacum officinale*) cools out liver excess symptoms and cleans up metabolic wastes in the blood.

Licorice (*Glycyrrhiza glabra*) a specific for peptic ulcers and constipation, it supports the adrenals.

Orange Peel (*Citrus*) a bitter digestive aid and stomach tonic, it's aroma imparts a fruity quality to the formula.

Cinnamon (*Cinnamomum cassia*) useful for passive bleeding from any mucous membranes, and stomach and gastrointestinal tract cramps.

Cardamon (*Elettaria cardamomum*) useful in gas and colic as a carminative.

Ginger (*Zingiber officinale*) for intestinal cramps and indigestion; a blood mover with warming properties for those with cold extremities.

MOTHER'S CORDIAL *This pleasant tasting compound syrup first appeared in the U.S. Pharmacopeia in the early 1900's and in 1922 in H.W. Felter's The Eclectic Materia Medica, Pharmacology and Therapeutics as a prepartum preparative for the last month of pregnancy to childbirth. It has been used for women who have had a difficult previous labor with difficult cervix dilation and women who have terminated early pregnancies. These herbs work synergistically to increase blood circulation and nutrients to the uterus and increase lymph drainage of waste products from that area, keeping tissues toned and nourished. Clinically, it increases the reactivity and sensitivity to oxytocin and decreases the prostaglandin threshold making it good for poor uterine tendon tone.*

Partridge Berry (*Mitchella repens*) tones and nourishes the uterus; allowing an easier childbirth.

Black Haw (*Viburnum prunifolium*) eliminates false or early labor pains.

False Unicorn (*Chamaelirium luteum*) is a uterine stimulant.

Blue Cohosh (*Caulophyllum thalictroides*) increases oxytocin, making contractions productive.

Cinnamon (*Cinnamomum cassia*) is a hemostatic, good for passive bleeding.

Vodka, Honey

NEUTRALIZING CORDIAL *This traditional formula is used in gastrointestinal crankiness due to either chronic constipation or crampy diarrhea; poor dietary metabolism with stomach ache, gas and sulphur burps due to fermentation. It will help in giardia and one-celled critters contracted from bad water. 1/2 to 1 tsp. for diarrhea; 2 to 3 tsps. for constipation.*

Chinese Rhubarb (*Rheum officinale*) used specifically for heartburn, acid stomach, and red pointed tongue (stomach heat), normalizing digestive pH.

Cinnamon (*Cinnamomum cassia*) soothing to the stomach membranes, reducing inflammation and drawing out heat.

Golden Seal (*Hydrastis canadensis*) good for excess mucus in the stomach and preulcerous conditions, cleaning and healing a sluggish or overactive system.

Peppermint Oil - an anti-microbial and aromatic disinfectant for stomach fermentation that accompanies gas and bloating.

Fructose, Ethanol (food grain), Vodka, Potassium Carbonate

OILS

EAR OIL *This oil has a soothing action on earaches and will help to loosen excess wax. One should warm up oil first. 2-3 drops is sufficient, use piece cotton ball to act as cork.*

St. John's Wort Oil, Mullein Oil, Garlic Oil

ARNICA/ST. JOHN'S WORT OIL *This massage oil soothes aches and pains in tight muscles, torn ligaments, bruises and spinal cord injuries as an anti-inflammatory to muscles and nerves innervating them. Useful in massage and rolfing sessions.*

CALENDULA/MULLEIN FLOWER OIL *This delicate light oil improves skin quality by increasing elasticity and firmness. It contains anti-bacterial properties and acts as a body oil, with special application to dry, cracked skin areas.*

ORGAN SYSTEM DISORDERS

This section gives a generalized synopsis of health problems and the traditional herbal remedies for them, categorized by the organ system and has been written specifically for the lay person with little or no herbal training. This information may be too general for individual pathologies. Diet, exercise and stress levels play a major role in dis-ease. Herbs can act as facilitators in the healing process. Many times these herbs are meant as adjunct therapies along with other compli- mentary modalities. For these and other more serious problems consult a clinical herbalist or naturopath.

RESPIRATORY – *sinuses, throat & lungs*

ASTHMA
   Humid – Elecampane, Horehound, Yerba Mansa, Yerba Santa, Grindelia, Breathe Deep
   Dry – Inmortal, Pleurisy, Lobelia

BRONCHITIS – Oshá-Wild Cherry Syrup, Eucalyptus (steam inhalant), Throat Spray
   Acute – Breathe Deep, Echinacea, Slippery Elm
   Chronic – Elecampane, Spikenard, Prickly Ash, Horehound, Grindelia
   Dry – Inmortal, Pleurisy

COUGHS – Oshá-Wild Cherry Syrup, Slippery Elm, Red Clover (children), Grindelia, Wild Cherry, Horehound-Marshmallow Syrup, Throat Spray
   Dry Irritative – Oshá, Lobelia, Pleurisy

HAY FEVER – Aller Aid, Nettles, Echinacea, Natural Resistance

HEAD COLD – Inmortal, Yerba Mansa, Ginger, Natural Resistance

INFLUENZA – Spikenard, Oshá, Natural Resistance, Echinacea, Yerba Mansa, Propolis, Eucalyptus or Thyme (steam inhalant), Throat Spray
   With Aches and Pains – Black Cohosh

LARYNGITIS – Slippery Elm, Marshmallow, Horehound-Slippery Elm Syrup, Throat Spray

PHARYNGITIS – Golden Seal, Echinacea, Red Root, Myrrh Gum, Gum Toner (as gargle), Throat Spray

SINUSITIS – Echinacea-Oshá Recipe, Inmortal, Yerba Mansa, Golden Seal, Ma Huang (use with care), Mormon Tea, Eyebright
   With Green Discharge – Baptisia, Grindelia

SORE THROAT/STREP THROAT – Gum Toner (to gargle & swallow), Red Root, Echinacea, Slippery Elm, Throat Spray

TONSILLITIS – Red Root, Oshá, Golden Seal, Yerba Mansa, Echinacea, Myrrh Gum, Throat Spray
   Chronic – Baptisia

GASTROINTESTINAL – *mouth, esophagus, stomach, small and large intestines*

CANKER (MOUTH) SORES – Echinacea, Dandelion, Burdock, Gum Toner
   Topical – Myrrh Gum (swish)

COLIC (CRAMPS) – Peppermint, Wild Yam, Catnip-Fennel Formula

COLITIS (CHRONIC) – Peppermint Oil Capsules, Marshmallow, Echinacea

CONSTIPATION – Cascara Sagrada, Bitter Tonic

DIARRHEA – Neutralizing Cordial, White Oak Bark

DYSENTERY – Quassia, Chaparro Amargosa, Neutralizing Cordial

GASTRITIS (INFLAMED STOMACH) – Marshmallow, Calendula

GASTRO ENTERITIS – Marshmallow, Yerba Mansa, Neutralizing Cordial

HEMORRHOIDS – Cascara Sagrada, Bitter Tonic
Topical – Shotgun Salve

HERPES – Yerba Mansa, Motherwort, Burdock
Topical – Golden Seal, Yerba Mansa, White Oak Bark, Propolis

HICCOUGHS – Peppermint, Black Haw

INDIGESTION (DYSPEPSIA) – Neutralizing Cordial, Gentian, Bitter Tonic

HEARTBURN – Blue Vervain

GAS – Cinnamon, Catnip-Fennel Formula

NAUSEA – Ginger, Wild Yam, Nausea Calm

PARASITES –
Pinworms – Black Walnut, Garlic
Giardia – Black Walnut, Quassia, Chaparro Amargosa

PEPTIC ULCERS – Marshmallow, Licorice

PYORRHEA/GINGIVITIS –
As Gargle – Myrrh Gum, Gum Toner, Bayberry

STOMACH FLU – Oshá, Echinacea, Marshmallow, Neutralizing Cordial

TOOTH ACHE –
Topical – Clove Oil

VOMITING – Chamomile, Mint, Wild Yam

LIVER AND GALLBLADDER

CHOLECYSTITIS – Fringetree, Celandine, Yarrow

CHOLELITHIASIS (GALLSTONES) – Celandine, Fringetree, Wild Yam

CIRRHOSIS – Milk Thistle, Celandine, Licorice

HEPATITIS – Milk Thistle, Fringetree, Licorice

JAUNDICE – Milk Thistle, Oregon Grape Root, Barberry, Fringetree, Dandelion

HEART AND BLOOD VESSELS

ARTERIOSCLEROSIS – Hawthorne, Ginkgo, Garlic, Lecithin, Devil's Claw, American Ginseng

HYPERTENSION – Hawthorne, Yarrow, Passion Flower, Garlic, Circula-Flow

HYPOTENSION – Hawthorne, Circula-Flow, Licorice

PALPITATIONS – Hawthorne, Motherwort, Circula-Flow

VARICOSE VEINS – Collinsonia, Ginkgo, St. John's Wort, Horse Chestnut
Topical – Witch Hazel

ENDOCRINE/METABOLIC – *adrenals, thyroid, pancreas*

ADRENAL EXHAUSTION – American Ginseng, Siberian Ginseng, Licorice, Ginseng-Licorice Formula

DIABETES/HYPERGLYCEMIA – Brickellia, Matarique, American Ginseng, Blueberry, Burdock

HYPERTHYROID – Bugleweed, Motherwort

HYPOGLYCEMIA – American Ginseng, Devil's Club, Cayenne, Prickly Ash

HYPOTHYROID – Gotu Kola, Oregon Grape, Passion Flower, Virginia Snake Root

OBESITY – Maravilla, Chickweed, Nettles, Guarana, Kola Nut

IMMUNE/LYMPHATICS

FEVERS – Echinacea, Elder, Yarrow

INFECTIONS – Echinacea, Myrrh Gum, LMPH Flow, Natural Resistance

    Fungal – Usnea, Canda-Tonic, Pau D'Arco, Desert Willow

MONONUCLEOSIS – Echinacea, Usnea, Red Root, Ocotillo, Cleavers, LMPH Flow, Immune Support

SUPPRESSION – Astragalus, Reishi, Burdock, Virginia Snake Root, Baptisia, LMPH Flow, Rejuvenation, Immune Support

REPRODUCTIVE

AMENORRHEA (suppressed menses) – Pennyroyal (do not use oil), Wild Ginger, Cotton Root Bark, Blue Cohosh, Dong Quai

CANDIDA – Pau D'Arco, Desert Willow, Usnea, Chaparral, Echinacea, Canda-Tonic

CERVICITIS – Raspberry, Partridge Berry, Dong Quai, False Unicorn, Calendula (douche), Echinacea (suppository)

CRAMPS (dysmenorrhea) – Blue Cohosh, Dong Quai, Wild Yam, Cramp Bark, Black Haw

CYSTS – Red Root, Chaparral, Dong Quai, Cleavers

ENDOMETRIOSIS – Chaste Tree berry, Black Cohosh, Pre-Mensease

FIBROIDS – Red Root, Ocotillo, Chaste Tree berry

IRREGULAR PERIODS – Menses Helper, Raspberry, Dong Quai (during estrogen phase), Chaste Tree (during progesterone phase)

MENOPAUSE – Dong Quai, False Unicorn, Meno Vitapause

PMS – Chaste Tree berry, Motherwort, Passion Flower, Pre-Mensease

PROSTATITIS – Saw Palmetto, Yerba Mansa, Dong Quai, Male Vitality

VAGINITIS – Echinacea, Yerba Mansa (sitz bath), Black Cohosh

SKIN, HAIR, EYES AND EARS

ABSCESSES (infection) – Echinacea, Cleavers, Yellow Dock

    Topical – Calendula, Comfrey, Shotgun Salve, Tea Tree Oil, Thuja

    Fungal – Usnea, Myrrh Gum

ABRASIONS –

    Topical – Shotgun Salve, Propolis, Myrrh Gum, Plantain, Comfrey

ACNE – Oregon Grape root, Yellow Dock, Dandelion, Burdock, Clear Skin

BALDING – **Topical** – Dogbane rinse, Jojoba oil

CONJUNCTIVITIS – Eyebright, Golden Seal (as saline eye wash)

ECZEMA – Burdock, Cleavers, Oregon Grape root, Devil's Club, Pleurisy, Clear Skin

    Topical – Grindelia

HERPES – Golden Seal, Yerba Mansa, Calendula, Oat seed, St. John's Wort, Dong Quai (genital)

    Topical – Simplex – Echinacea, Myrrh Gum

    Genital – Yerba Mansa (sitz bath)

INSECT BITES – **Topical** – Echinacea, Shotgun Salve

OTITIS MEDIA (middle ear infections) – Eyebright

POISON IVY/OAK – **Topical** – Plantain, Grindelia, White Oak Bark, Itch Away

PSORIASIS – Burdock, Yellow Dock, Cleavers, Oat seed, Clear Skin

TINNITIS (ringing in the ears) – Pulsatilla, Ginkgo

TIRED EYES – Blueberry, Eyebright, Bright Eyes

NERVOUS SYSTEM AND PAIN

ANXIETY – Motherwort, Pulsatilla, Mellow Out

DEPRESSION – St. John's Wort, Passion Flower, Lift the Spirits

INSOMNIA – Passion Flower, Skullcap, Hops, Valerian, Sleep Easy

MENTAL SLUGGISHNESS – Ginkgo, Gotu Kola, Creativity

NEURALGIA – Skullcap, Black Cohosh, St. John's Wort, Mellow Out

PAIN
 General – Black Cohosh, Prickly Poppy, Valerian, Aspen
 Hangover – Oregon Grape root, Guarana, Chaparral, Toadflax
 Sciatica – Skullcap
 Headaches – Skullcap, Clematis, Feverfew, Valerian, Guarana, Passion Flower, Feverfew-Clematis Compound
PARALYSIS – Oat seed
 Topical – fresh Cow Parsnip

URINARY TRACT

CALCULUS (STONES) – Shepherd's Purse, Gravel Root

CYSTITIS/URETHRITIS – Yerba Mansa, Agrimony, Pipsissewa, Urisoothe
 Chronic – Uritone, Buchu, Juniper

INCONTINENCE – Corn Silk, Horsetail, Agrimony

PAIN – Marshmallow, Kava, White Willow, Aspen, Corn Silk, Wild Yam

MUSCULO-SKELETAL *(includes connective tissue)*

ARTHRITIS – Devil's Claw, Yucca, Limber Up, Nettles

BRUISES/SPRAINS, BREAKS – Black Cohosh, Comfrey
 Topical – Arnica, St. John's Wort

GOUT – Shepherd's Purse, Devil's Claw

RHEUMATISM (myalgia) – Black Cohosh, Angelica, Echinacea, Devil's Claw, Feverfew, Limber Up
 Topical – Wintergreen or Eucalyptus oil

TENDONITIS/BURSITIS – Echinacea, Prickly Ash

PRE/POST PARTUM (OBSTETRICS)

ANEMIA – Nettles, Yellow Dock

LABOR FACILITATORS – Black Cohosh, Blue Cohosh, Inmortal, Cotton Root bark

LACTATION – Alfalfa, Fennel, Cotton Root bark, Blessed Thistle, Mother's Milk Flow

MASTITIS – Cotton Root bark, Red Root, Echinacea

MORNING SICKNESS – Peppermint, Nausea Calm Wild Yam

PREPARATUS – Mother's Cordial, Raspberry

SITZ BATH – Uva Ursi, Yerba Mansa (saline)

STRETCH MARKS – Calendula & Mullein oil mas

THREATENED MISCARRIAGE – Cramp Bark, Black Haw, Wild Yam

CHILDREN

COLIC – Anise, Chamomile, Catnip-Fennel Formula

CRADLE CAP – Thuja, Tea Tree oil

DIAPER RASH – Marshmallow powder, Shotgun Salve

DIARRHEA – Fireweed & Peppermint tea

EAR INFECTIONS – Ear oil, Echinacea, Mullein oil

ERUPTIVE DISEASES (Chicken Pox, Measles, Mumps)– Echinacea, Yarrow, Natural Resistance for Kids
 Topical – Witch Hazel

FEVER – Echinacea, Elder, Yarrow, Pansy, Natur Resistance for Kids

HEADACHE – Burdock, Skullcap

HYPERACTIVITY – Motherwort, Calm-A-Kid, Chamomile, Hops, Kid's Focus Power

IMPETIGO (Thrush) – Topical – Usnea wash
 Internal – Usnea

TEETHING – Chamomile, Passion Flower, Clove (diluted)

VOMITING – Lavender, Peppermint, Slippery El (gruel)

REFERENCES & SUGGESTED READING

American Herbalism: Essays on Herbs & Herbalism by Members of the American Herbalists Guild, Crossing Press, Freedom, CA 1991

Direct Marketing Registry of Ethical Wildcrafters & Organic Growers of Medicinal Herbs, Rocky Mountain Herbalist Coalition, P.O. Box 165, Lyons, CO 80540

Earth-Validated Offerings of the Rocky Mountain Herbalist Coalition: Deep Green Herbal Activism Comes of Age, 1992 RMHC

Eclectic Materia Medica, Pharmacology & Therapeutics, H.W. Felter, Eclectic Medical Publications, Sandy, OR, 1922

Foundations of Health, the Liver & Digestive Herbal, Christopher Hobbs, Bonanica Press, Capitola, CA, 1992

Gathering the Desert, Gary P. Nabhan, University of Arizona Press 1985

Green Pharmacy, The History and Evolution of Western Herbal Medicine, Barbara Griggs, Healing Arts Press, Rochester, Vermont 1981

Healing Wise, Susun Weed, Ash Tree Publications, Woodstock, NY 1989

Herbal Medicine, R.F. Weiss, M.D., Beaconsfield Publishers Ltd., Beaconsfield, England 1985

Herbal Repertory in Clinical Practice, Michael Moore, Southwest School of Botanical Medicine, PO Box 4565 Bisbee, AZ 85603

Holistic Herbal, David Hoffman, Findhorn Press, Scotland 1983

Kings American Dispensatory, Vol. I & II, Felter-Lloyd, Eclectic Medical Publications, Sandy, OR 1983

Medical Botany, Lewis/Elvin-Lewis, Wiley-Interscience, NY, NY 1917

Medical Herbalism, A Clinical Newsletter for the Herbal Practitioner, P.O. Box 20512, Boulder, CO 80308

Medicinal Plants of The Desert & Canyon West, M. Moore, Museum of New Mexico Press, Santa Fe, NM 1989

Medicinal Plants of the Mountain West, M. Moore, Museum of New Mexico Press, Santa Fe, NM 1979

Medicinal Plants of the Pacific West, Michael Moore, Red Crane Press, Santa Fe, NM 1993

Matura Medicina and Naturopathic Dispensatory, Kuts & Cheraus, American Naturopathic Physicans and Surgeons Assn., Des Moines, Iowa, 1958

The Male Herbal, James Green, Crossing Press, Freedom, CA 1991

Therapeutic Herbalism, Correspondence Course on Phytotherapy, David Hoffman, Sebastopol, CA

ADVANTAGES OF DIFFERENT PREPARATIONS

Tinctures are a preferred form for bitter medicinals; the taste can be disguised in juice or sweetened tea. Tinctures provide quick assimilation and ease of administering dosage. Many herbs contain glycosides, alkaloids and resins that may not give up their medicinal properties to a water base such as teas and many herbs in loose bulk form cannot be guaranteed of freshness. Tincturing the fresh or freshly dried plant is a sure method of stabilizing the shelf life of an herb as the alcohol acts as a preserver. The term 'extract' can mean any strength, but tinctures are USPS standardized ratios of 1:5 herb to liquid with anywhere from 40 to 95% alcohol as the prescribed medium. 15-20 drops of extract is equivalent to a #0 capsule; 25-30 drops is equivalent to a #00 capsule.

Teas or medicinal infusions also have certain advantages, particularly if one cannot tolerate even the slightest amount of alcohol. Hot teas of diaphoretic herbs stimulate sweating relatively fast. Larger amounts of vitamins, minerals and enzymes can be extracted with longer steeping of nutritional water soluble herbs. Also teas are relatively inexpensive.

Capsules, if freeze dried, will probably contain high quality plant material. Dried ground herbs will lose some properties if the plant is volatile but will contain non-water soluble constituents.

CALCULATIONS OF DOSAGES FOR INFANTS AND CHILDREN

Herb dosages for children can be calculated by using Clark's rule.

Clark's Rule: Divide the weight (in pounds) by 150 to give the approximate fraction of the adult dose. For example, a 50 pound child will require 50/150 or 1/3 the adult dose.

It is important to understand that the above calculation gives only approximate dosages and that individual requirements may vary widely. Also, young children may be very susceptible to certain herbs or relatively unsusceptible to others. If ever in doubt as to the proper use or dosage of an herb, the advice of a qualified herbal practitioner should be sought.

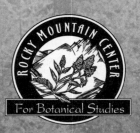